A More

Beautiful
You

A More
Beautiful

You

*Reverse Aging
Through
Skin Care,
Plastic Surgery,
and Lifestyle
Solutions*

Robert M. Freund, M.D., F.A.C.S.

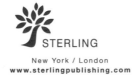

STERLING

New York / London
www.sterlingpublishing.com

STERLING and the distinctive Sterling logo are registered trademarks
of Sterling Publishing Co., Inc.

Library of Congress Cataloging-in-Publication Data Available

10 9 8 7 6 5 4 3 2 1

Published by Sterling Publishing Co., Inc.
387 Park Avenue South, New York, NY 10016
© 2010 by Robert M. Freund, M.D., F.A.C.S.
Distributed in Canada by Sterling Publishing
c/o Canadian Manda Group, 165 Dufferin Street
Toronto, Ontario, Canada M6K 3H6
Distributed in the United Kingdom by GMC Distribution Services
Castle Place, 166 High Street, Lewes, East Sussex, England BN7 1XU
Distributed in Australia by Capricorn Link (Australia) Pty. Ltd.
P.O. Box 704, Windsor, NSW 2756, Australia

Sterling ISBN 978-1-4027-5628-3

For information about custom editions, special sales, premium and
corporate purchases, please contact Sterling Special Sales
Department at 800-805-5489 or specialsales@sterlingpublishing.com.

SPRINGER & SISTER
Produced by Springer & Sister
www.springerandsister.com

Interior design by Mary Springer

To my loving wife, Judy,
and our four adorable kids,
Jake, Ben, Emily, and Jonah

Thank you for your patience and understanding

CONTENTS

ACKNOWLEDGMENTS

Thank you to Drs. Joel Kassimir, Ron Brancaccio, and Lance Brown for their assistance in making the dermatological parts of this book current and interesting. Thank you to the best cosmetic dentists—Drs. Ken Fishman, Steve Roth, and Timothy Chase—for their advice on everything related to cosmetic dentistry.

A special thanks to the Diet Diva, Kerry Gans, for making "Beauty Food" the best regimen for looking and feeling good. Thanks to Felicita T. Rada and Bianka Lefferts for their expertise on all things related to hair care and to Susan Ginsberg for her help with makeup.

Thanks to Aimee DeGrazia, Shelly Mattachione, and Bibi Hemraj for technical support and hard work at keeping a busy office running while I was busy putting this work together.

Thanks to Susu Langlands for her help on the manuscript and Lauren Cosentino for her excellent artwork.

Finally, thanks to my parents, Paula and Harold, for their guidance and support.

INTRODUCTION

It was my first day as an attending plastic surgeon. Fresh from the rigors of a tough training program, I was confident, knowledgeable, and certain that I could handle any plastic surgery or beauty question that came my way. Although I had treated more than one thousand patients during my residency, for the first time I had no safety net, no senior authority figure to turn to. Yes, I could always call a trusted mentor to discuss a difficult case, but I could hardly waste my colleagues' time with ordinary procedures. What's more, if I were to reveal my insecurity by consulting on something routine, I feared their loss of confidence in me—an absolute no-no!

But more important than all of the knowledge I had acquired, even more important than all my hard-won surgical skills, was that I was wearing the requisite pinstripe suit of a plastic surgeon. You see, plastic surgeons strive to present an image a step above the ordinary white-coat look worn by most respected doctors. Plastic surgery is all about the hype, or at least that was what I was led to believe.

As a resident, I heard stories of famous plastic surgeons hiring models to sit in the waiting room of their nascent practices when prospective clients came calling. This maneuver serves several purposes. First, it tells the patient that their doctor is important enough to have a model as a client. It is a common assumption that models have an inside track to the very best in plastic surgery. Forget for a second the fact that models are beautiful not because of their brains or analytical skills, but because they are born with one essential asset and that is good genes!

The second reason for the models' presence is to make patients feel even more insecure about their particular concerns than when they came into the office. Put yourself in the patient's seat, looking across at this beautiful person. Although you may have come in to see the doctor to have a mole removed, once you see the model's beautiful lips, your lips are not looking so good. When you go in to see the doctor, you cannot resist, and before you know it, you're getting some filler to plump up your lips. For the doctor, the investment of a model in the waiting room is starting to pay off!

Finally, having a beautiful woman in the waiting room is a testament to the fine surgical skills of the physician. If she looks good, you will look good, too! This line of reasoning may remind you of a cosmetic advertisement or a commercial for some wonderful new shampoo. Big companies rely on beautiful models or celebrities to sell their boring shampoo that is no different than a thousand other shampoos on the market. These companies want you to believe that by using their shampoo, you will look like the beautiful young model with perfect hair who was primped and propped for four hours prior to the photo shoot. Needless to say, neither a shampoo nor a plastic surgeon can deliver on such an unrealistic expectation.

So, back to my first day as an attending: I walked into the consultation room and proceeded to take my patient's medical history and perform a precise medical exam. To me these steps were essential. After many years of hard training, I still considered myself a physician and, in the end, the ultimate goal was the medical care of the patient. As I went through my questions and exam, the patient, let's call her Pam, studied me with a quizzical look. She told me that she had been on three previous consultations with other doctors and, in each case, the exam was cursory. In one doctor's office, Pam remembers speaking with a prescreener (a nurse or physician's assistant) who did a brief exam and provided minimal description of her options. The physician then strutted into the room with office staff in tow, claiming to have all the answers to Pam's concerns. The only way for a physician to make a confident diagnosis is to perform a thorough exam. Secondhand reporting of a patient's physical findings yields secondhand results. In the end, Pam received little in the way of alternatives or benefits. How was she to feel comfortable in that type of office? Well, it is a lot like the almighty Oz. If the hype is large enough, then small details such as risks, alternatives, and benefits may be lost in the hoopla.

In another office, Pam met with a surgeon who highlighted her weaknesses and made her feel worse about herself than she had when she walked into the office. She was so distraught during this encounter that she began to cry. As a young surgeon, new to this game of plastic surgery hype, I was at a loss to explain why the doctor would behave that way. Yet, over time, I came to realize that one trick of the trade is to exacerbate the insecurities of your patient. As her insecurity grows, so will her desire for a surgical procedure—or so the conventional thinking goes. In my view, my job as a plastic surgeon is not to promote a patient's insecurity, but to study the insecurity to determine its origin and decide if a plastic surgery procedure is appropriate.

This point deserves emphasis. Many patients come to me to correct a deformity that is making them self-conscious and uneasy. For most people the level of concern is proportional to the physical findings. For a small group, however, the patients' emotional responses to their "deformity" are disproportionate to the severity of the problem. This latter group is stricken with a psychological disorder called body dysmorphic disorder, and for this group, surgery should be avoided at all costs. The problem of body dysmorphic disorder is discussed further in chapter 14, Teens and Cosmetic Surgery.

Common sense suggests avoiding people who make you feel bad about yourself, and this holds true in the plastic surgeon's office as well. Of course this tactic is not limited to plastic surgeons. Salespeople at the cosmetics counter of your local department store may be trained to point out shortcomings and then profess to have the miracle cream to save the day. I'll discuss this more in chapter 4, Beauty in a Bottle.

In the third doctor's office, Pam recounted how the doctor told her about deformities and signs of aging that even Pam had not considered. Although she went to the doctor looking for advice concerning her lips, that doctor without solicitation advised her about issues of many other parts of her face and then proceeded to describe the multiple surgical procedures that Pam would need to rectify the problems. The problem with this third doctor's advice was that the only thing that bothered Pam was her lips. This is akin to a woman asking her husband if a dress looks good on her and in response he says that she looks fat and that her makeup is awful. Obviously, these types of interactions do not work well for either the patient or the physician. Yet, some doctors act more like car salesmen than physicians.

So, back to our interview. I had now gotten a basic understanding of Pam's health history and concerns regarding her face. At that point, I proceeded to describe her options and discuss the risks, as well as what she could expect from our treatments. I told her almost everything I knew about the lips, and felt like the consultation was going well. However, that's when things got difficult. You see, Pam then started to ask about skin care and other things that she could do to enhance her looks and slow the aging process. I dismissed those topics. I thought that discussion of nonsurgical procedures was beneath my position as a plastic surgeon.

I could not have been more wrong. As I now know, some of my bluster was based on a lack of training when it came to prevention and skin care. At the time that I came out of my residency in plastic surgery, quality skin care and prevention of aging were not considered important aspects of plastic surgery as they are now. As you will see in chapter 3 on dermatology and chapter 4, Beauty in a Bottle, prevention and other types of skin care are now seen as the first critical line of defense against aging. With this in mind, you can see how important this facet of medicine is to plastic surgeons. If my goal is to provide the best aesthetic results for my patients, then these topics should always be part of my treatments.

Another reason for my avoidance of these treatments as part of my armamentarium was the invisible line that separates plastic surgeons from dermatologists. Plastic surgeons often regard themselves as above any treatment that another physician may also prescribe, such as the fillers or other skin remedies employed by dermatologists. Now, there are many plastic surgeons who refer their patients to dermatologists for routine maintenance, me included. However, this does not eliminate my responsibilities as a doctor to understand all the associated treatments to my specific organ system. To make it clear, I am not suggesting that all plastic surgeons should know the intricacies of the kidneys or the lungs, only that they should understand everything regarding the skin. Conversely, I hope that dermatologists, as the other key provider of aesthetic health care, also take it upon themselves to understand the basics of plastic surgical alternatives so they can appropriately advise their patients in this regard.

And so it began, my quest to understand all the components of my patients' care that, in spite of being well trained as a plastic surgeon, I had little knowledge of. As my efforts began, I culled various resources to try to decipher fact from fiction. This is where a science background is essential. At all levels of cosmetic health care, hype tends to overwhelm science. To this point I have described how plastic surgeons can get caught up in the hype, but that is only the beginning. Some dermatologists and plastic surgeons have started to sell products called cosmeceuticals in their office. As their name suggests, cosmeceuticals are a hybrid product somewhere between pharmaceuticals (strong and effective with FDA oversight) and cosmetics (an unregulated topical product that is more camouflage than effective skin care). Despite the wonders claimed by these cosmeceuticals, they are still only a modestly effective cousin to real pharmaceuticals that are designed to treat and improve your skin.

Is there an ethical dilemma created when so many physicians now sell cosmeceuticals in their offices? Some critics would say that a doctor has a moral obligation to be a physician first and not a salesman for fancy moisturizers. To those critics, I would argue that although these products are not much different than anything available over the counter at your neighborhood pharmacy, a benefit is provided in finding a professionally selected group of products at your physician's office. Furthermore, physicians can draw upon feedback from patients, so each of the products they sell will have been tested in everyday use. Of course, this reasoning is only as good as the physician who takes the time to research and evaluate the products he or she provides. There will always be those unscrupulous doctors who try to sell you whatever they have in stock, despite your lack of interest, desire, or need.

As my indoctrination into the fraternity of plastic surgeons continued, I was troubled by the problem of aesthetics. "What is beauty?" may seem like an easy question at first glance, but upon further consideration it isn't so. Often throughout my residency, I wondered if the procedures I performed made the patient more beautiful or just not as wrinkled. Surprisingly, the ideals of beauty were not a subject of discussion at any level in my training. The old adage "beauty is in the eye of the beholder" has some truth to it; what is beautiful to one person may not be so to others.

So, what can I tell my patients about beauty that will help them make educated decisions about which treatments they choose to receive? Chapter 1, What Is Beauty?, will set you on the first part of your journey to *A More Beautiful You*. This chapter will describe different definitions of beauty throughout the ages as well as from different societies. Researching the literature to gain a better understanding of beauty has helped me in evaluating my own patients and ultimately formulating a better surgical plan to enhance each one's beauty.

After leaving my residency training program, it was clear that my understanding of treatments to help prevent and treat fine lines, photoaging, and blemishes was lacking. As is to be expected, the emphasis was on surgery, not topical creams and potions. The chief of our department, who often shunned any interest in anything related to cosmetics, best exemplified this. This is partly due to the fact that plastic surgery has a proud history as a reconstructive field (the first kidney transplant was performed by a plastic surgeon). Many also prefer to emphasize the more "noble" aspects of plastic surgery, such as correcting children's congenital deformities or cancer-related reconstructions, over cosmetic surgery.

Now, as a plastic surgeon who practices in the aesthetic arena, I have dedicated a significant amount of my time to learning about topical products that can help my patients, both before and after surgery. Many of these same medications that are used by my plastic surgery patients can also be used by almost any person interested in keeping his or her skin healthy and protected from the ravages of the sun and pollution. Chapter 2, Skin Health and Skin Care, will develop your understanding of what makes up your skin and how to protect and rejuvenate it. This chapter will define the basics of anatomy as well as the factors that ravage your skin over time. I will also discuss some of the different treatments that have been created to reverse the aging process.

Chapter 2 will also discuss skin care products available over the counter. It may interest you to know that the majority of products available at your local drugstore are just glorified moisturizers surrounded in hype. Companies resort to beautiful models and celebrities to pitch their products as the greatest thing since sliced bread, regardless of their merits. These highly paid endorsers often see, smell, and feel the product for the first time when they enter the studio to say how great it is! Labeling of these products is also full of hype. Many key phrases on the packaging sound convincing but mean little.

In the past 15 years, cosmetic dermatology has grown by leaps and bounds. Originally dermatologists focused only on diseases of the skin. Over time, their knowledge was brought to bear on treatments for beautiful skin as well. Dermatologists have been pioneers in the many treatments now available for your skin. Facial wrinkles and other signs of aging can be treated effectively with fillers or Botox. FDA-regulated pharmaceuticals are available for preventive skin care that are very effective and require a doctor's prescription. In chapter 3 you will bypass much of the hype and learn about nonsurgical treatments that actually have some effect.

Going beyond protecting your skin and keeping it healthy, I would like to set you on your way to looking as beautiful as possible. Imagine your face as a beautiful picture, with the shape of your nose, the pout of your lips, and the tilt of your eye all making up your own unique portrait. With this in mind, a better frame will high-light key features of the picture just as your hair frames your face. Chapter 5 will discuss hair and makeup and ways to enhance your natural beauty while avoiding common pitfalls.

Part Two of this book will focus on the distinct areas of your face and the surgical treatments available to help you look more beautiful or just a little rejuvenated. The chapters are broken down into regions that are affected by each particular treatment. For example, in chapter 6, on the lower face, I will go into the varied treatments that help correct sagging of the cheeks and neck. This is a logical progression because the unique procedures available to both those areas are often the same.

Chapter 7 will discuss the eyes, eyebrows, and forehead. Although these anatomical areas are often treated at the same time as the lower face, the assortment of treatments available merits separate consideration. Chapter 8, on the nose, will discuss all the ins and outs of probably the most difficult component of cosmetic plastic surgery. Chapter 9 will consider the mouth and teeth, with a complete discussion of plastic surgery of the lips as well as dental treatments and surgery. Chapters 10 and 11 cover procedures for the ears and hair, respectively.

Once you have a basic understanding of the science and art of plastic surgery, it is time to decide whom should you consult with to determine if plastic surgery is right for you. As with any big decision, getting the right advice is essential to a good result.

Plastic surgery is unique in the medical field in that it may be the only time that you may submit to surgery when you are not sick. Let's think about that for a second. Say you have a bulge on your abdomen that is diagnosed as a hernia. A hernia can be a life-threatening problem and, as such, your general surgeon suggests that you have corrective surgery. If you do not like what your surgeon is telling you, you can certainly see another doctor, but the likelihood is that doctor will also suggest a corrective procedure to repair the hernia.

Cosmetic surgery is different, because whether or not you have surgery is up to you. You will be healthy before the surgery and hopefully you will be healthy after the surgery. But the underlying concern is that you will be subjecting yourself to the risks of surgery and anesthesia for a procedure that is not strictly medically necessary. To increase the odds of a successful outcome, you will certainly want to find the best doctor for you, who may or may not be on the list of top doctors in each specialty that crops up annually in your local paper. For advice on finding the best plastic surgeon for your needs, see chapter 12.

Now that you have chosen the right surgeon and the time is drawing near for your surgery, there are certain things that you can do to prepare yourself for the big day and help with your postsurgical recovery. Chapter 13, on presurgical preparation and postsurgical recovery, will help you have the best and easiest recovery.

There are many sources of concern in our society that influence the self-image of our children. Hollywood constantly highlights an image of perfect features and slim figures. Is it any wonder that eating disorders are so prevalent in our society? As a concerned parent, I often wonder if these issues will plague my own children. Now you may say that as a physician, I have access to a magic wand to ensure that problems of adolescent self-image will not affect my own children, but you could not be further from the truth. As a parent, I make many mistakes along the way. Love and concern are the best remedies I can prescribe.

We have all heard stories of teenagers who try to correct their emotional issues through plastic surgery. How is a parent to decide if their child wants or needs plastic surgery for the right reasons? On the other hand, as a caring parent, shouldn't I offer my children an option such as plastic surgery so they can feel good about themselves? Well, turn to chapter 14, Teens and Cosmetic Surgery, to get a simple guide to dealing with your children and their adolescent demons.

As a whole, *A More Beautful You* delivers a crash course in beauty. The book was conceived to bring together the varied, often confusing, sources on the different aspects of beauty and provide an all-encompassing primer. I further set as a goal of the book to provide all the latest up-to-date options for each facial concern as well as an unbiased comparison of the many options.

Quite often, women come to my office looking for help after their last child leaves for college. These patients typically describe a life dedicated to children, carpools, and late nights helping their children succeed. Through it all, Mom was typically last in line for care and consideration. Now that her last child is gone, she takes a deep breath, looks in the mirror, and comes to the realization that although the years have passed by quickly, her skin and facial features have counted each and every moment of those difficult 20 years.

Now for this hypothetical patient, I could outline all the different options for reclaiming some of the beauty lost over a 20-year journey of motherhood and leave it at that. However, the fun part of this job is that the majority of improvement and the changes in behavior necessary to carry those improvements forward can be enacted in a matter of weeks. With that in mind, the last chapter of the book is a guide to implementing all the best techniques for beauty and personal satisfaction in a mere 12 weeks. It may sound too good to be true. Perhaps for some who have experienced the excessive ravages of the sun or smoking improvements may be limited, but with my knowledge based in science, not hype, I am most certain that almost anyone (men included) can benefit from 12 weeks on my program.

Finally, I set out on this quest to provide the ultimate beauty bible only after I felt comfortable with my knowledge and understanding of the many options available to you, the consumer. With memories of my uncertainties on that first day as an attending plastic surgeon, only now do I feel adequately prepared to tell this story and dispel the myths and hype, while enlightening my readers about all the great options at hand. So without further ado, I invite you to begin the journey to *A More Beautiful You.*

PART ONE

Foundations of
Beauty

Chapter 1

WHAT IS BEAUTY?

"Love of beauty is Taste. The creation of beauty is Art."

—Ralph Waldo Emerson

We have all heard the expression "beauty is in the eye of the beholder." And while some may find this a somewhat naive, though well-meaning, sentiment, it does underscore a critical point. Despite centuries of examination and thought, a simple definition of beauty continues to elude us. In eras past, philosophers, poets, painters, and even mathematicians tried answering the question of what makes a person beautiful. Today it seems we are still trying to figure it out.

The image-saturated world in which we live offers a constant bombardment of supermodel perfection, making the rest of us mortals feel as if we can never measure up. But is that really the definition of beauty to which we should aspire? Should people base their sense of self on the airbrushed, blemish-free world of glossy magazines—a world whose sole purpose is to sell us things?

As a cosmetic surgeon, my life's work has been to make people more physically attractive, so I am not about to say that outer beauty does not matter. But I firmly believe—and many social studies support this belief—that a person's beauty is more often than not determined by her physical attributes *in conjunction with* her personality traits. Being overly concerned about conforming to a strict ideal of physical perfection does not really guarantee you anything except a lighter wallet and a lot of disappointment.

To some readers it may seem odd that I am writing a book about how to become more beautiful while proposing that a perfect ideal of beauty is hard to define. It shouldn't.

Early in my career I came to understand that each one of my patients had a slightly different idea of what would make him or her more beautiful. And this made me realize that, in the end, the concept of beauty is actually very human: slightly imperfect, considerably subjective, and unendingly complex.

This chapter will explore the reasons why it is so difficult to arrive at a definition of beauty to satisfy everyone. Attractiveness is a personal judgment based on a combination of three things: a few universals that have been determined by our evolutionary history, the prevailing norms of our own culture, and each individual's subjective preference.

In trying to understand what is truly beautiful, I hope that I will put you on the path to discovering you own beauty—both inner and outer—and how to best maximize it.

BEAUTY AND OUR EVOLUTIONARY HISTORY

The idea of beauty as we know it does not exist in the animal world. Rather, innate cycles of courtship, mating, and caring for offspring repeat themselves *ad infinitum* to ensure the continued survival of each species. However, even though the behaviors are innate, there are certain physical qualities that do help the natural processes along.

It has been well documented that animals are attracted to symmetrical qualities when looking for a mate. For example, female swallows prefer males with more symmetrical tails, and female zebra finches seek out mates with symmetrically colored leg bands. Beyond mating, studies have shown that, given a choice, human infants show a preference for staring at symmetrical faces rather than asymmetrical ones. In the animal world, symmetry is an important determinant in assessing overall health and strength. For example, a horse with symmetrical legs will run faster than one with asymmetrical legs, making it more likely to survive when fleeing a predator.

Youth and "cute," infant-like features are also considered attractive. Austrian zoologist Konrad Lorenz theorized that physical features such as small body size, large eyes, a small nose, dimples, and round, softer bodies trigger a nurturing response in adults, which, in turn, helps ensure that offspring grow to adulthood and procreate. Scientific studies have shown that infant-like, "cute" physical qualities (big eyes, small nose, and a clear complexion) are universally accepted as attractive across the globe.

What do these attributes have to do with our human ideals of beauty? Because the qualities of symmetry and cuteness influence mate selection, they have, through the process of evolution, encouraged the continuation of species. And this common evolutionary history with animals has carried over to humans, affecting what we deem desirable and beautiful. Although our finely tuned ideals of beauty vary from culture to culture, these few basics—having been genetically programmed by our evolutionary history—are universal.

BEAUTY AND PREVAILING CULTURAL NORMS

Once we move beyond the unchanging universals of beauty (symmetry, health, youth, and infant-like features), the attempt to classify what is attractive becomes much more difficult. Would a woman in sixteenth-century France be considered beautiful by today's standards? How about an Eskimo man trying to woo a Nigerian woman? Would she find him attractive in the same way the women back home do?

A person considered beautiful in one culture is by no means guaranteed the same reaction in another. Just as we are influenced by our evolutionary history, so too does the society in which we live shape what we deem beautiful. And this changes over time. For example, women considered attractive in the early 1900s had rounder, fuller figures than their counterparts in 1968.

Anyone reading this book is probably well aware of the current prevailing norms of beauty in our culture—they are pervasive. And they do affect us as a society. "Lookism," which is discrimination based on perceived attractiveness, abounds. Studies have shown that good-looking students get higher grades, handsome criminals get lighter sentences, and overweight people make less money. And for those of you who appreciate a bit of schadenfreude, lookism can operate in both directions. For example, it has been shown that beautiful women have fewer female friends because of hostility, jealousy, and distrust toward them.

Jokes aside, it can be quite demoralizing if you do not fit the prevailing societal norm of beauty. Neverthless, each one of us has a unique look that should be embraced and maintained. Is reducing the size of an overly large nose a good idea? Of course. Would getting rid of the sagging skin around your neck make you look younger? No doubt. Yet, as I tell all my patients, it is important to beware of getting too caught up in what society defines as beautiful. Beauty is not simply soulless imagery—it comes to life through much more than just your physical features.

BEAUTY AND OUR OWN SUBJECTIVITY

We have all heard the snide comments: "He is such a good-looking guy. He could have married anyone and he ended up with that plain Jane!" Or, "What is that loser doing with her? She is so gorgeous." While these comments are cruel, they are also illuminating, for two reasons. First, they perpetuate the falsehood that the only thing that matters, above all else, is the way someone looks. Second, and more important, they illustrate that very often physical appearance is not the determining factor when choosing a partner—contrary to the billions of dollars spent trying to convince us otherwise.

Beauty *is* in the eye of the beholder. When people meet, there is a sizing up that occurs, a subjective interpretation of the other person. Physical attributes will certainly be considered, yet even those will be viewed through an individual lens. Some people might find a larger man handsome, while others prefer women with curly hair. And though these may not represent prevailing cultural norms, they do not stop anyone from finding such physical attributes attractive.

Personality comes into it as well. Traits like intelligence, charm, grace, humor, self-confidence, and empathy are part of the overall impression made by a person. One study showed that 70 percent of college students deemed an instructor physically attractive when he acted in a friendly manner, while only 30 percent found him attractive when he was cold and distant.

The bottom line is that physical perfection is not the way to find personal fulfillment, to create successful relationships, or to have a lucrative career. It is the combination of both inner and outer beauty that makes a person truly attractive.

BEAUTY AND THIS BOOK

I believe you should use all of the tools at your disposal to make yourself as beautiful as possible. But I also think it is critical to understand that no matter which options you choose, none will come with a magic wand able to suddenly make your life perfect.

To see through the pervasive hype that surrounds the beauty industry, you need to approach it in an educated, methodical, and rational manner. It is my hope that this book will help you do just that. From over-the-counter remedies to surgical procedures, you will learn everything you need to know to make the right choices—choices that will work for you.

It is my firm belief that everyone has the potential to be a truly attractive person. But remember that this overall impression of beauty includes your personality as well as your physical appearance. And while I can't offer advice in the personality department, I can make certain you know everything you need to know to make yourself more physically attractive.

So let's get started!

Chapter 2

SKIN HEALTH AND SKIN CARE

"Like anyone else, there are days I feel beautiful and days I don't, and when I don't, I do something about it!"

—Cheryl Tiegs

The only time we think of our skin is when there is a problem. Whether we have wrinkles, loss of elasticity, or uneven skin tone, the effects of aging are right there for everyone to see. It can sometimes feel like a cruel trick of nature that the most exposed skin—that of our face—is the most prone to the ravages of the sun and time. Yet, despite what may seem like a losing battle, there are things you can do to keep your skin looking young and healthy. Remember that knowledge is power, so the more you know about your skin—its anatomy, regenerative processes, and basic chemistry—the better able you will be to protect it.

The skin, which is your body's largest organ, performs a variety of important functions essential to maintaining overall good health. It acts as a protective barrier against bacteria and other toxic elements, it helps insulate you from both heat and cold, and it gets rid of toxins in your body through perspiration. Your skin also tends to prominently display signs of aging, especially on your face. The good news is that paying close attention to your lifestyle choices, adhering to a healthy diet, and choosing the right products can effect improvements in the appearance of your skin. The even better news is that you can actually repair damage that has already been done.

Before going any further, it is important to note that doctors classify the aging of your skin in two ways. The first is chronological, and this is just as it sounds—the skin of a woman in her seventies will have certain characteristics (less elasticity and decreased thickness, for example) based on nothing else but her age. The second is called photoaging and is determined exclusively by exposure to harmful UV rays of the sun, which causes skin to become leathery, wrinkled, and blotchy. A 22-year-old can actually have skin that is more aged than a 52-year-old, for example, simply because of their differing exposure to the sun. A simple way to illustrate this point would be to compare the facial skin of a frequent sunbather with the protected skin below her bikini line—the difference would be dramatic. The fact that doctors even have to distinguish between these two types of aging should be enough to send everyone running to buy sunscreen and a big floppy hat. It cannot be overstated: Unprotected exposure to the sun ages you faster and more noticeably than your actual years do!

In order to implement an effective strategy to slow the signs of aging, you will need both a basic understanding of how your skin functions and an awareness of the things you are trying to protect against. Sun is obviously "enemy number one," but there are many other factors to consider. Even where you live can affect how your skin looks! I am not suggesting that you move to a less-polluted area, but I use this example to emphasize an important point—the more you know about what effects your skin, the more options you will have to improve your appearance.

ANATOMY

The three layers that comprise your skin are the epidermis, the dermis, and subcutaneous tissue.

EPIDERMIS

Epidermis is the layer of skin that is visible to the naked eye. It acts as a protective shell, helping to keep toxins, bacteria, and viruses out of your body. Your epidermis,

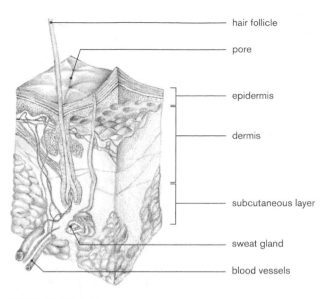

hair follicle

pore

epidermis

dermis

subcutaneous layer

sweat gland

blood vessels

LAYERS OF THE SKIN

Epidermis is the thin top layer of skin. The dermis is the thick middle layer with hair follicles, sweat glands, and blood vessels. The subcutaneous tissue is made of fat, blood vessels, and the connective tissue that holds everything together.

which is constantly renewing itself, is made up of two layers—the basal layer and the stratum corneum. The basal layer consists of live cells that, as they move toward the surface, die and become part of the stratum corneum. These dead cells then flake off, a process that can be accelerated with the use of various exfoliating techniques. As the live cells move closer to the surface they build up large amounts of keratin, which further strengthens the epidermis. Pigment cells, which determine your skin color, are also found in this top layer of skin.

DERMIS

Located directly below the epidermis, the dermis is the real "workhorse" of your skin. It contains nerve endings, hair follicles, sweat glands, and blood vessels, forming a connective tissue that provides structure to your skin. The two critical proteins of your skin—collagen and elastin—are found in the dermis layer. Both of these proteins, when subjected to the effects of aging, will adversely alter the way you look. A loss of collagen weakens the overall structure of your skin, causing it to look thin and paper-like, while a loss of elastin lessens the ability of your skin to return to its original position, similar to what happens when the elastic band in your underwear loses its elasticity.

The area where the epidermis and dermis meet, while not a separate layer, is worth mentioning because it is important to your overall skin health. This dermal–epidermal junction provides a way for your epidermis to receive nutrients from the blood vessels located in the dermis. Rete ridges, which act as small bridges between the two layers, reach out from the dermis into the epidermis, enabling the outermost layer of skin to benefit from the flow of nutrients in the blood. When this flow is constricted, your epidermis will suffer. Factors that affect the blood supply include stress, pollution, smoking, and the sun.

SUBCUTANEOUS TISSUE

The bottom layer of skin is made up mostly of fat cells. These cells act as both insulators and volumizers. Thus, the loss of fat cells as you age can affect your ability to stay warm as well as make you appear a bit hollowed-out. Subcutaneous tissue also has small fibers, called fascial bands, that connect the underlying muscles to the skin. If these bands stretch out, the skin will sag.

All three layers of your skin will age chronologically, eventually showing signs of cellular and DNA damage. But if that were the end of the story I would not be writing this chapter, nor would skin creams, peels, exfoliants, and supplements be a thriving multibillion-dollar business. The operative word in the first sentence is "chronologically." Yes, we all age—albeit some better than others—and we have to accept that. Yet there are ways to slow the aging process as well as to guard against premature photoaging.

THE BASICS OF PREVENTION

In addition to sun exposure, there are many other lifestyle variables responsible for premature aging. And while these factors may seem widely divergent, they have one thing in common—the ability to damage your skin on the cellular level. Cigarette smoke (both first- and secondhand), excess alcohol, pollution, stress, an imbalanced diet, and lack of sleep can wreak havoc on your skin, causing wrinkles, discoloration, a dry, dull texture, and loss of elasticity.

If you are serious about staving off the signs of premature aging, start paying attention to those things you have control over. Adopting positive changes to your diet, sleep habits, and alcohol consumption are just as important as quitting smoking. And, of course, protecting yourself from the sun's harmful rays goes without saying! But what about those things you cannot control, like secondhand smoke and environmental toxins? Is there anything you can do to protect your skin from these?

Before examining specific lifestyle cause-and-effect relationships (how improving the nutrition of your diet can improve your skin quality, for example), it is a good idea to learn what can go wrong with your skin at the cellular level. With better understanding you will be better able to make the right choices for overall skin health.

FREE RADICALS AND ANTIOXIDANTS

No doubt you have heard the terms *free radicals* and *antioxidants* a lot over the past 15 years. The discovery of free radicals and their action in the body began quite apart from any dermatological connection. Free radicals were initially studied to understand their relationship to the injury of the blood vessels in patients with high cholesterol or a history of smoking. It wasn't until the 1990s that the cosmetics industry began to see a connection between free radicals, antioxidants, and skin health. Since then, the scientific community has learned how free radicals damage your skin and what effective steps can be taken to prevent this damage.

Each cell in your body needs oxygen to survive, including your skin cells. A free radical is a damaged oxygen molecule that has only one electron in its outer shell instead of two. The laws of nature dictate that this damaged oxygen molecule will scavenge electrons from other molecules in order to replace its missing electron. This in turn causes a chain reaction of scavenging, threatening the stability of the entire cellular structure. The damage is even more pronounced if the electron is taken from the DNA, because it can cause a break in the strands of cellular information. With this disruption, the cell will stop operating properly and run the risk of becoming prematurely old or, worse, cancerous.

If the science sounds a little complex it might help to imagine a ballroom dance. Let's say there are 15 couples moving gracefully across the floor when suddenly one partner twists an ankle and must stop dancing. Feeling embarrassed to be standing alone, the remaining partner cuts in on one of the other couples, which in turn leaves that partner alone, who then cuts in on another couple. All of sudden, what had been a nicely choreographed dance is now unstable and thrown into disarray. In essence, this is what happens to your cells when free radicals are on the loose. Unlike a dance, this molecular instability can weaken your overall health, so it is no laughing matter.

Antioxidants are molecules that do not become destabilized upon losing an electron, and thus are able to break the negative chain reaction of scavenging. By introducing antioxidants into the system, the free radicals are neutralized because they are now stealing from molecules that will not scavenge to replace their lost electrons. Going back to our ballroom dancing metaphor, it would be as if there were a substitute to take the place of the injured partner so as not to disrupt the remaining pairs of dancers.

Unchecked free-radical damage to your skin usually results in premature wrinkles, fine lines, and sagging skin. This damage is caused when cell function is compromised, activating enzymes called metalloproteinases that break down your skin's collagen and elastin. With less collagen and elastin your skin is not able to repair itself and will become thinner and less resilient and take on a more leathery appearance. Beyond the appearance of wrinkles (which we can live with even if we would prefer not to), free radicals can damage your skin to the point that it becomes more prone to serious disease such as skin cancer.

I should point out that we all have free radicals in our system. Under normal circumstances our bodies fight them with enzymes designed to counteract the effects of free radicals from normal stores of vitamins C and E. But the aging process, UV radiation from the sun, smoking, and pollution diminish both the amount and the effectiveness of our bodies' own antioxidants. And once the ratio of free radicals to antioxidants becomes too high, excessive damage can occur.

There are three ways to increase the amount of antioxidants available to help keep your skin looking young: eating foods that are rich in antioxidants, taking vitamin supplements, and using topical treatments that contain antioxidants. All three—done in the proper way—have proven to be surprisingly effective in neutralizing the damage of free radicals.

The three main antioxidants are vitamin C, vitamin E, and beta-carotene, which is a form of vitamin A.

Vitamin C. This water-soluble vitamin is found in most citrus fruits as well as bell peppers, broccoli, cauliflower, and leafy greens. Studies have shown that vitamin C is particularly effective in protecting against free-radical formation due to cigarette smoke and pollution. The recommended daily allowance (RDA) is 60 mg, but you can take up to 1,000 mg a day. Anything above 2,000 mg may cause unwanted side effects in some people, so you should experiment and find the right daily dose for your own particular body. The best oral form of vitamin C is Ester-C, which is more bioavailable than other forms. Bioavailability refers to the degree to which a substance is absorbed and able to be used by the body's systems. Vitamins with high bioavailability stay in your body and do not flush out of your system through your urine. For creams, topical vitamin C should be in the L-ascorbic acid form only, which enables it to penetrate to the dermis layer. It should also have a concentration of at least 20 percent or it doesn't have much effect. Keep in mind that L-ascorbic acid degrades when exposed to sunlight, which is why antioxidant vitamin C creams such as Cellex-C are packaged in dark bottles.

Vitamin E. This fat-soluble vitamin is found in vegetable oils, nuts, seeds, fish oils, olives, spinach, asparagus, whole grains, and fortified cereals. Vitamin E is considered extremely effective in stopping the chain reaction of electron-stealing free radicals in your body and should be thought of as the primary defense against oxidation. Since the recommended daily requirement for vitamin E is hard to achieve from food alone, it is a good idea to take a supplement. The current RDA is 15 mg per day for men and women over 14 years old. That may be low, but be careful not to exceed 400 IU (1 mg of alpha-tocopherol is equivalent to 1.49 IU of the natural form or 2.22 IU of the synthetic form) per day, as reports show that higher doses may increase your risk of heart disease or cancer. It should be pointed out that these findings have received some criticism because the studies focused on only one type of vitamin E (d-alpha-tocopherol, which is prevalent in multivitamins). To err on the side of safety, try to find a vitamin E that includes at least eight types of tocopherol or tocotrienol. Of additional concern to doctors is that vitamin E is fat soluble and does not flush out of the body with urine, so excess amounts may end up stored in your liver. Thus, while vitamin E is an extremely effective antioxidant, it is important to use moderation when taking it.

Beta-carotene. There is no RDA for beta-carotene because it is converted to vitamin A by your body. This essential nutrient is found in spinach, yams, liver, butter, cantaloupe, egg yolks, milk, carrots, tomatoes, grains, and peaches. You can only get beta-carotene in foods, so there is no risk of overdoing it. You should be aware that vitamin A in supplement form is not an antioxidant and can be toxic at high levels.

Beyond vitamin C, vitamin E, and beta-carotene, there are other antioxidant creams and supplements being marketed as the next magic bullet in the fight against aging. Idebenone (sold as Prevage cream), proanthocyanidin (sold as RevaléSkin cream), as well as the supplements resveratrol, coenzyme Q10, omega-3 fatty acids, and alpha-lipoic acid are all sure to have some positive effect on your cells, including those of your skin. But the science surrounding this field is still new, so exaggerated claims—which are often reprinted in the nonmedical press—should be met with some skepticism.

While antioxidant topical creams will be discussed in greater detail in chapters 3 and 4, two caveats need mentioning here. First, be careful that the active ingredient concentration is not too high, because this can cause skin irritation. A simple test is to apply the antioxidant cream behind your ear several nights in a row, and then watch to see how you tolerate the cream. Second, these creams and gels will not be particularly effective unless they reach the lower layers of the skin. Thus, their ability to be absorbed will determine their usefulness. The only way for you to be sure that this is happening is to apply them after cleansing your skin, but before any other creams or lotions are applied.

For those whose eyes glaze over when trying to understand which foods to consume and in what amounts to foster better skin health, the Diet Diva, Keri Gans, and I have formulated a one-week eating regimen that maximizes the best foods essential to preserving healthy and youthful-looking skin. Let's be clear that Beauty Food is not a diet. I am of the belief that most diets eventually fail, because of the inherent deprivation necessary for diets to succeed. Beauty Food is a framework for healthy living. To see how Beauty Food works, go to appendix A, and start eating to support your beauty today.

beauty food

THINGS TO AVOID

Now that you have a basic understanding of what happens to your skin on a cellular level, we can return to the real world of lifestyle choices. As mentioned earlier, your skin ages in two ways—chronologically and prematurely due to bad habits. While it goes without saying that as you get older your skin will show signs of aging, it can only help to incorporate healthy habits into your daily regimen sooner rather than later. In fact, some studies conclude that a large amount of photoage damage is done before the age of 20! Of course, for many of us it is too late to turn back the clock and avoid those mistakes. But remember that your skin reacts well to being taken care of properly and is actually capable of repairing some of the earlier damage that occurred. So it really is never too late to get started.

Sun. There is really nothing worse for your skin than prolonged, unprotected exposure to the sun's damaging rays. UVA rays (ultraviolet "aging"), which are present throughout the year during all daylight hours, penetrate more deeply and affect the dermis. UVB rays (ultraviolet "burning") are present during the summer months at peak midday hours and affect the epidermis. Damaging effects of the sun include deep and excessive wrinkles, leathery or dry skin, discolorations, and a weakened immune system. While the exact reasons as to why the sun is so bad for your skin are still not fully understood, we do know that it stimulates enzymes (metalloproteinases) that break down your skin's collagen and elastin stores, increases free radicals in your body with potential injury to the DNA of the cell, and disrupts the rejuvenation processes of your skin cells.

An increased risk of cancer is probably the most compelling reason to protect yourself against the sun. Research has shown that exposure to sunlight can release chemicals in your body that interfere with the ability of your white blood cells (T lymphocytes) and specialized skin cells (Langerhans) to attack developing cancer cells. The free radicals that are created by UVA rays can also cause genetic defects that may start a cell on the path to becoming cancerous. Additionally, UV exposure can interrupt the natural process of apoptosis (when damaged cells die) by allowing them to live, divide, and possibly become cancerous.

Cigarette Smoke. As everyone knows, smoking is terrible for you and can lead to a variety of life-threatening diseases, so it is hard for me to believe that anyone still smokes. But since people do, it is worth noting that smoking also causes severe premature aging to your skin in a variety of ways. First, research suggests that smoking produces higher levels of the enzymes called metalloproteinases, which can break down your skin's collagen and elastin. These enzymes can also damage your DNA, causing sun spots and skin cancer. Second, smoking significantly decreases the moisture in your skin, leading to more wrinkles. Third, cigarette smoke causes a reduced flow of blood to the skin, which allows more free radicals to be created and disrupts your skin's ability to regenerate properly. Fourth, the constant presence of tar and nicotine in the mouth area predisposes smokers to a higher risk of lip, mouth, and throat cancers (those who chew tobacco are also at risk for these types of cancer). Finally, some studies have hypothesized that distinct "smoker" wrinkles form around your mouth and eyes due to the repeated muscle movement of taking a drag and squinting from the smoke in your eyes. All of which add up to five more reasons you should not smoke!

Alcohol Consumption. While an occasional glass or two of red wine (an important source of resveratrol) is not harmful, any alcohol in excess may cause premature aging of the skin. Alcohol is a source of free radicals, it can destroy your body's supply of vitamin A (an important antioxidant), and it dehydrates your skin, causing a dull, dry complexion. Keeping your alcohol consumption to a minimum can help in achieving your goal of healthy, young-looking skin.

Stress. Being under stress puts enormous pressure on your entire body, including your skin. Chronic stress produces high levels of adrenaline, which cause a restriction of blood flow and allow more toxins to build up. Adrenaline also stimulates the production of cortisol, which retards skin regeneration.

Lack of Sleep. If, due to stress or other factors, you are not getting enough sleep, your cortisol levels will rise. Cortisol is a steroid hormone that controls many different systems in your body. Too much cortisol retards skin regeneration during the nighttime hours, when regeneration should be at its highest. It follows logically that if a lack of sleep prevents your skin from regenerating properly, you are going to look older. So as Ben Franklin said, "Early to bed, early to rise, makes a man healthy, wealthy, and wise." I think it is now appropriate to add "younger-looking" to that list!

Pollution. While no one would expect you to move to the countryside in order to protect your skin against premature aging, you can take steps to lessen the effects of pollution if you live in a city. Carbon monoxide and sulfur dioxide are two pollutants that affect blood flow to the skin. Since both are most prevalent at rush hour and on hot days, it is best to try to limit your time outdoors during those times, especially if you are planning to go out and exercise. Installing HEPA filters in your house or apartment can help get rid of some toxins and pollutants in the air. Finally, pollution effects the strength of the sun, making it more dangerous because of the depletion of the protective ozone layer—yet another compelling reason to wear sunscreen.

PREVENTATIVE MEASURES

Now that I have defined the problem and the factors that can contribute to prematurely aging your skin, what are the true solutions to mitigating their effects? Every day we are bombarded by advertisements that promise a reversal of the aging process. While some methods are tried and true, others are merely the latest buzzwords of the cosmeceutical industry. The following steps will help you mitigate the effects of aging without breaking the bank.

USE SUNSCREEN

Even if you avoid midday sun and wear protective clothing, sunscreen is still necessary to keep you safe from the harmful effects of UV rays. With so many products on the market, it is hard to know which ones are the most effective. Before I get into the specifics there are a few things that need mentioning. Sunscreens should be water resistant even if you do not plan to swim—this ensures that you won't perspire it off. Sunscreens should also be applied liberally and often regardless of their SPF. Keep in mind that the use of sunscreens is probably one of the few times when too much of a good thing *is* a good thing!

There are two general types of sunscreens—chemical and physical. A chemical sunscreen absorbs UV rays, while a physical sunscreen reflects the harmful rays away from your skin, like a temporary coat of armor.

What offers the best protection? Recent studies have shown that physical sunscreens are the safest and most effective choice. First, they block both UVA and UVB rays, which most chemical sunscreens do not. Second, physical sunscreens are active the moment they are applied, while chemical sunscreens require time (typically 30 minutes) to absorb into your skin. Third, some people may find chemical sunscreens irritating to the skin, while physical sunscreens are not (the physical sunscreen zinc oxide is in most diaper creams, which are applied to extremely sensitive skin!). Fourth, reports suggest that some chemical sunscreens (avobenzone) deteriorate rapidly in the sun. Finally, there are some findings that show chemical sunscreens may actually create free radicals, the exact opposite of what anyone wants a sunscreen to do. Applying an antioxidant cream before a chemical sunscreen can help, but with good physical sunscreens available that do *not* create free radicals, there's no reason to take a chance.

The most effective ingredient in chemical sunscreens is ecamsule (Mexoryl SX) because it is the only one that blocks both UVA and UVB rays, offering you broad protection. Ecamsule is currently available in Anthelios, a moisturizing sunblock made by La Roche-Posay. However, ecamsule does not provide broad-spectrum UVA protection and therefore avobenzone is added to the sunblock to provide more coverage. The problem with avobenzone is its high rate of decay in the sun, which renders it ineffective rather quickly. The best physical sunscreen is zinc oxide, especially now that there is a new micronized formula that is clear—no more embarrassing bright white noses! And, since physical sunscreens are not absorbed into the skin, they have not been found to create free radicals, making them the current top choice for sunscreens.

Sunscreens are available labeled with a sun protection factor (SPF) ranging from 2 to more than 100. Any SPF higher than 15 or 20 is overkill. In fact, these products can be a bit dangerous in that they lull you into thinking you are so protected you may forgo other important preventative measures like wearing a hat or sitting under a

	Active Ingredient	UVA Block	UVB Block
chemical sunscreens	avobenzone (Parsol 1789)	broad coverage	none
	cinnamate	none	limited
	ecamsule (Mexoryl SX)	limited	none
	octocrylene	none	broad coverage
	oxybenzone	limited	yes
	PABA	none	limited
	padimate O	none	limited
	methyl anthranilate	limited	none
	homosalate	none	limited
physical sunscreens	zinc oxide (including micronized)	best coverage	yes
	titanium dioxide	good coverage	yes

beach umbrella. SPF ratings are based on the assumption that unprotected skin starts to become damaged after only 15 minutes in midday sun. The SPF rating represents the length of time you will be protected, expressed as a multiple of "safe" 15-minute blocks. Therefore, a lotion with an SPF of 20 allows for five hours in the sun, while an SPF of 60 allows for 15 hours in the sun (a highly unlikely scenario unless you are in Finland in June). Again, there is nothing intrinsically wrong with high-SPF sunscreens, I just worry that they may lead to reckless behavior, actually causing more skin damage than if you were wearing none at all!

Because of confusion in the current sunscreen labeling system, in the next year the FDA has advised the industry to change to a new labeling standard. First, SPF ratings will measure the protection against UVB rays only. Second, a new four-star system will be instituted for rating UVA protection (with one star signifying the lowest protection and four stars signifying the highest protection). Finally, sunscreens will now only be categorized as water resistant or highly water resistant. Companies will no longer be allowed to label sunblocks as "waterproof"—which none truly are.

EAT A HEALTHY DIET

As you have already learned, antioxidants are important to protecting your overall health, as well as your skin. Luckily, many of the foods that we eat are rich in antioxidants. Your goal should be to eat at least two to three servings each day of foods that can naturally provide your body with a strong defense against free-radical damage. Supplements are called "supplements" for a reason—they should be used to add to those vitamins you are already getting from your diet, rather than being the primary source of these important nutrients.

Antioxident	Food Sources
vitamin A	liver, eggs, carrots, spinach
vitamin C	broccoli, bell peppers, oranges, spinach
beta-carotene	carrots, broccoli
vitamin E	vegetable oil, nuts, green leafy vegetables
omega-3 fatty acids	walnuts, salmon, flaxseed oil, soybeans

Eating foods that are rich in nucleic acid offers another relatively painless antiaging strategy. Foods such as salmon, shellfish, lentils, beans, chickpeas, mackerel, and sardines have been shown to lead to an increase in your body's production of adenosine triphosphate (ATP), a nucleotide that is critical to the basic functioning of your cells. While the science is still out on this, some believe that more ATP can provide your cells with improved energy and a stronger ability to regenerate. Whether or not this theory pans out, eating a lot of lentils and shrimp certainly cannot hurt, so incorporating foods that are rich in nucleic acid into your diet is a good idea.

Staying well hydrated is also an important part of staying healthy and is key to keeping your skin young-looking. Try to drink at least eight glasses of water a day. Green tea and citrus juices have the added benefit of providing you with a great source of antioxidants while keeping you hydrated.

REDUCE STRESS AND SLEEP MORE

While these two goals may sound straightforward, they are probably the most difficult to achieve. Most of us lead busy lives with many pressures that are out of our control. Getting by on meager hours of sleep and feeling constantly stressed out are the status quo. And, since both are now widely accepted, we have lost sight of how truly damaging these habits have become. Recent studies show that chronic sleep deprivation is more detrimental to your health than being overweight or not exercising. Stress is also terrible for your body—and your skin. Among other things, both inhibit your ability to rejuvenate on a cellular level and all the consequences that come with that.

Use this book to take stock of your lifestyle and try as hard as you can to incorporate more healthy habits. Even if you are lucky enough to be naturally good-looking, you will not radiate beauty when you are not taking care of yourself. So the first step in any beauty regimen is to actually strengthen your health. Getting more sleep is a step in the right direction, as is utilizing various stress-reducing strategies such as yoga.

NEW AGE MEDICINE

The above information on skin—and the aging process—is based on newer science that focuses on cellular machinery, the study of which has provided doctors with improved tools in handling these issues. Recently, some doctors calling themselves "New Age" physicians have taken this science to another level. While much of their philosophy and resulting recommendations falls in line with generally accepted medical practices, some treatments have become very controversial—for good reason, which will be explained below.

This area of research is still in its beginning stages. Tinkering with your body's chemistry in any sort of extreme way is a risk—especially when the long-term benefits of doing so have yet to be proven. Throughout this book my medical advice will always be moderate and err on the side of caution. That is not to say that "safe" translates into minimal results—it does not. Rather, practicing medicine responsibly based on peer-reviewed science means I am not putting my patients at risk even as I rejuvenate them. Not all New Age physicians can say that.

The following is a brief summary of the main goals of New Age medicine and how these relate to your skin.

Restore antioxidant levels to reduce free radical levels. Although many of these physicians say they understand the optimal level of antioxidants for each and every individual, I find this hard to believe. Antioxidant levels necessary to maintain a healthy body vary from person to person and minute to minute. In addition, these optimum levels change as we age. New Age practitioners are very often proponents of high levels of antioxidants. However, most mainstream medical professionals suggest moderate levels that are supplementary rather than corrective. This more cautious approach takes into consideration that extreme amounts of antioxidants can become pro-oxidants and do more harm than good. The best way to achieve a moderate intake of antioxidants is through eating foods rich in vitamin C, vitamin E, and beta-carotene, primarily fruits and vegetables, as discussed above.

Decrease the glycation of proteins by controlling serum glucose levels. Western diets typically include too much sugar, and this excess sugar in our bloodstream can bind to our proteins. When this happens, the aging process of the proteins is sped up, which negatively impacts the structures they create. No one would disagree that too much sugar in a diet is a bad thing. Rather, the controversy starts when deciding how to correct the problem. The generally accepted practices of low-glycemic diets, exercise, and using supplements to control glycation (including alpha-lipoic acid, vanadium, chromium, zinc, and taurine) have been shown to work. However, New Age physicians take this a step further and suggest using prescription drugs formulated for patients with diabetes (either Glucophage or metformin) to control blood sugar elevations in otherwise healthy patients. Needless to say, prescribing such strong medications for patients who are not sick is seriously unconventional and could carry risks that have yet to be properly understood.

Maintain an optimal level of proteins in the bloodstream. This strategy is designed to provide the building blocks for tissue regeneration. Increasing the protein in your diet is relatively easy to accomplish and presents no controversy. It is also a good idea to increase meal frequency so that you are eating small amounts every three to four hours.

Create an optimal ratio and quantity of fatty acids. This is important because the fatty acids act as building blocks of cell membranes that control blood flow, inflammation, and hydration. New Age medicine proponents also suggest controlling the inflammatory process with a low-allergen diet supplemented with lactobacillus, amino acids, and omega-6 and omega-3 fatty acids.

Ensure the needed supply of cofactors for tissue growth and regeneration. Cofactors are molecules that aid the function of other molecules in the body. Without them, the growth and regeneration of your body is slowed. As well as the usual list of vitamins, cofactors include CoQ10, alpha-lipoic acid, magnesium, calcium, and selenium.

Reduce the detrimental effects of cortisol. As mentioned earlier, cortisol can negatively affect your skin's ability to regenerate. Cortisol can be reduced by increasing meal frequency, incorporating relaxation techniques into your life, and getting enough sleep.

The last two objectives of New Age medicine are the most controversial.

Restore steroid hormone levels such as estrogen, testosterone, DHEA, and progesterone. It is no secret that the hormonal changes associated with aging affect the entire body, including outward appearance. For example, many women will attest to the fact that as menopause sets in, elasticity and thickness of the skin reduce quite dramatically. This is no coincidence: Estrogens play a key role in the look and health of your skin; as these hormones decline, so does your skin's quality. In the past, hormone replacement therapy proved to be a great way to counteract this. However, more recent studies have shown that there may be risks to taking these medications.

An alternative to hormone replacement is phytoestrogens, which are plant-derived nutrients that mimic human estrogens. But evidence as to whether they work is still unclear, and they too present some serious issues worth considering. First, as these molecules circulate through your bloodstream, they not only mimic your own estrogens, but they also tell your body to stop making its own estrogens. This can severely reduce your estrogen stores, thereby eventually creating a situation where your body has no choice but to rely on these supplements for support. The second, and perhaps more important issue, has to do with estrogen regulation. Your body is a finely tuned machine, and the estrogen levels in your bloodstream are kept within tight control on a minute-to-minute basis. Therefore, it is wholly unrealistic to expect a supplement that you consume once or twice a day to be as well managed as your own estrogen levels. Overall, there has not been nearly enough study done on whether these types of supplements are able to manipulate estrogen levels properly or how they affect the rest of your body.

Restore growth hormone levels. Recent scandals in the professional sports world have reignited the debate over human growth hormone (HGH). While its proponents insist that HGH offers positive results, critics focus on what they consider to be the crux of the debate: At what cost? This is especially true regarding the long-term effects of

HGH on the body, because not enough time has elapsed to study it properly. Ironically, proponents of HGH are often most keen on its supposed ability to extend longevity! Studies do show that HGH can increase lean muscle mass, thicken the dermal elements of your skin, and increase skin elasticity, all of which sounds great. However, there is evidence that HGH also increases IGF-1, a growth factor that may be linked to cancer. HGH can also deform the bones of the skull and jaw. You may remember the professional wrestler Andre the Giant. Well, Andre had a condition that made his pituitary gland produce too much HGH. As a result, he had a prominent brow, enlarged jawbone, and a freakish overall giant look—not an aesthetic that anyone is keen to achieve.

The only current legal use of HGH is by people who suffer from demonstrable deficiencies in the hormone, about 7 percent of the general population. And as recent baseball scandals have illustrated, use of HGH by anyone else is illegal. Therefore, this new sector of the skin care market will remain off-limits to most of us for the time being—which is a good thing until more research is conducted. Avoiding HGH is a wise move for both your health and your wallet. The annual cost to a patient on growth hormone therapy is between $15,000 and $20,000. Even though its use is illegal, there are still plenty of unscrupulous doctors willing to break the law—and it is no wonder, considering the amount of money to be made.

Internet Resources: Suntan Lotions and Beauty Product Evaluation

www.ewg.org/whichsunscreensarebest/2009report

Chapter 3

COSMETIC DERMATOLOGY

"Dermatology is the only specialty in medicine where there are 200 diseases and only three types of cream to treat them."

—Anonymous

It used to be that a patient visiting the dermatologist's office had a case of acne, unexplained dermatitis, or concerns about skin cancer. Times have certainly changed! Of course, a dermatologist is still the specialist to see if you are dealing with any type of skin disease or problem. But over the past decade dermatology has shifted its focus, placing a stronger emphasis on cosmetic procedures and products rather than traditional medicine. As is the case with any change, there are pros and cons to the rapidly expanding cosmetic dermatology industry.

This chapter will provide you with the tools you need to navigate what has become quite a crowded marketplace. Like other facets of the beauty industry, cosmetic dermatology has its fair share of hype. But with a bit of knowledge, you can increase your chance of getting the most for your money and choosing the procedures and products that are right for you. Your dermatologist offers many effective ways to enhance your appearance—you just need to know how to separate fact from fiction.

Any discussion of dermatology must also include what has traditionally been its area of expertise: the diagnosis and care of skin diseases. Your skin is a complex organ, and any problem with it demands a skin specialist. So remember that even though dermatologists are now doing cosmetic procedures, they still represent an important part of your overall health care, especially when it comes to the early detection and treatment of skin cancer.

THE ANATOMY OF YOUR SKIN

As you may recall from chapter 2, your skin is made up of three main layers that keep your body hydrated, regulate its temperature, protect against external pollution and free radicals, create vitamin D from the sun, and excrete toxins from your body. They are the epidermis, dermis, and subcutaneous tissue.

The epidermis is the layer of skin that is visible to the naked eye. Dead cells in this layer usually just flake off. If not, they may begin to accumulate and your skin can look dull.

Located directly below the epidermis, the dermis layer provides for the thickness, elasticity, integrity, and strength of your skin. It is also where you will find nerve endings, hair follicles, sweat glands, and oil glands. The cells of the dermis are called fibroblasts. These cells are responsible for producing three critical components of your skin—collagen, elastin, and hyaluronic acid. Collagen, a protein, adds strength and substance to your skin, while elastin, another protein, gives your skin its ability to return to its original position after being stretched. Hyaluronic acid is a sugar that plays an important role in keeping your dermis hydrated.

Your epidermis receives nutrients from the blood vessels located in the dermis via rete ridges, which act as small bridges between the two layers. When this flow is constricted your epidermis will suffer. Factors that affect the blood supply include stress, pollution, smoking, and the sun.

Made up mostly of fat cells, the subcutaneous tissue layer is located below the dermis. These cells act as both insulators and volumizers. As you age, the loss of fat cells can affect your ability to stay warm as well as make you appear a bit hollowed-out.

EFFECTS OF AGING ON THE SKIN

The amount of collagen, elastin, and hyaluronic acid in your skin starts to diminish from the day you are born. And while fibroblast cells continually produce more of these three critical substances, at a certain point the aging process overwhelms the cycle. This weakens your skin's ability to regenerate properly. To add insult to injury, this decline is not just a matter of quantity; the *quality* of your skin's collagen, elastin, and hyaluronic acid diminishes with age as well. Thus, a three-year-old not only has more collagen but better collagen than her grandmother does.

Later in this chapter I will detail the many cosmetic products and procedures designed to mitigate the effects of these changes. But keep in mind that as you age your cellular machinery is slowing down, so there are limits to how much improvement can be made using cosmetic solutions alone. Cosmetic dermatological procedures and products are useful tools early on in the aging process, helping patients slow down the inevitable decline of their skin quality. It goes without saying that the sooner you start protecting and nourishing your skin, the better it will look at any stage of your life.

Contrary to popular belief, the fundamental mission of dermatology is not to make your skin look more beautiful. Rather, the top priority of any dermatologist is to first make certain that your skin is *healthy*. Once that has been established, then you are free to explore the varied options available to you in the growing field of cosmetic dermatology.

SKIN DISEASE

The three main types of skin problems that dermatologists diagnose and treat are acne, dermatitis, and skin cancer. If you are not interested in learning about acne and dermatitis, please feel free to skip ahead. However, I implore you to read the skin cancer section. We all tend to think that will never happen to us, but no one is immune from the possibility of skin cancer. And while you may be conscientious now, unprotected sun exposure when you were a lifeguard during the summer of 1984 can lead to your being diagnosed with cancer today. Early detection is a critical factor in survival rates for any type of cancer. The more you know about skin cancer, the better chance you will have of catching it in time for it to be treated properly.

ACNE

Although acne is typically associated with the hormonal changes of puberty, people of all ages can suffer from it. Acne is caused by the overproduction of oil that becomes "trapped" in the skin by clogged sebaceous glands in the dermis. This type of blockage can occur not only because of changes in hormone levels but also because of poor personal hygiene or heavy emotional stress.

Nonprescription creams and gels that contain benzoyl peroxide are usually an effective treatment for mild to moderate acne. If the acne persists, a dermatologist can prescribe stronger medication—either Retin-A or Accutane. Retin-A, a tretinoin, is a topical treatment that not only dries up the acne but also sloughs off the dead skin cells that are blocking the sebaceous glands. Retin-A comes in both cream and gel form. Some dermatologists recommend the gel because it is more drying, providing a slight edge in clearing up the acne faster.

Accutane, an isotretinoin that comes in pill form, is very effective in clearing up persistent acne. It works from the inside out by drastically reducing the production of oil from the sebaceous glands (as compared to Retin-A, which dries up the oil that has been produced). However, Accutane comes with a very high risk (90 percent) of causing birth defects if it is taken by pregnant women. This is obviously a serious concern since acne tends to present itself in teenagers—the same group that engages in unprotected sex and has high rates of unwanted pregnancies. Because of this risk, the FDA strictly regulates the prescribing of Accutane through the iPLEDGE program. Patients must sign a form, promising to use protection if they are sexually active while taking Accutane. However, this program has not done much to lower the incidence of pregnancy, so most dermatologists simply will not prescribe Accutane to teenage girls.

Accutane also impairs the healing of wounds, even if you have not taken it for a year. Therefore, it is essential to avoid any surgery while taking Accutane and for at least 12 months afterward.

Finally, laser technology has recently been touted as a promising new way to treat acne. The Isolaze, a machine that is both vacuum and laser, offers a multipronged approach to clearing up acne. The vacuum opens up the pores and then the laser cleans them out, killing bacteria as it does so. Studies have shown that lasers may offer short-term results; however, Accutane is still considered the best long-term treatment. As with most new products, I tend to err on the side of caution, especially when it involves directing beams of intense light at your face. Therefore, my advice would be to avoid laser treatments for treating acne until they have been in use long enough to fully understand their myriad pros and cons for this particular application.

DERMATITIS

This category covers a large array of skin disease. In fact, the category is so broad that it is impossible for us to cover it adequately within the confines of this chapter. Dermatologists have bookshelves full of volumes devoted to the causes and manifestations of dermatitis. For our purposes, it is sufficient to understand that conditions such as eczema, psoriasis, and seborrhea are outward signs of dermatitis and they are, generally speaking, some form of an inflammation.

Steroids are the best way to treat dermatitis. Over-the-counter steroids, such as cortisone creams, are a good place to start, but they may not be strong enough to get rid of the problem. Prescribed steroids can be administered as either a topical cream or a pill. Just keep in mind that—over time—steroids can both thin and dry out your skin. If the condition persists you and your doctor may want to reassess your treatment before the steroids do too much residual damage. If steroid treatment is not effective, there is a new group of medications called immune modulators that have been successful in treating inflammatory skin disorders, including psoriasis. These drugs have side effects but are worth exploring if other treatments have failed.

SKIN CANCER

There are three common types of skin cancer: basal cell carcinoma, squamous cell carcinoma, and malignant melanoma. Each varies in the way the cancer presents itself, how serious the risk to your health is, and what form of treatment is recommended. Since the sun is the main cause of the disease, skin cancer usually appears in the sun-exposed parts of your body. Genetics play a role as well. So if you have a blood relative who has had skin cancer you should be particularly vigilant about not only protecting yourself against the sun but also about having yourself screened annually. And, of course, everyone should use an effective sunblock 12 months a year.

Basal Cell Carcinoma. This is the least dangerous of the skin cancers, although it should still be taken *very* seriously. Basal cell carcinoma usually appears as a small, red lesion that may or may not be slightly raised. Very often the lesion has shiny white edges around it that dermatologists refer to as "pearly." Sometimes the lesion can be ulcerated and bleed, resembling an open sore. Basal cell skin cancer is locally invasive, meaning that it will very rarely spread to other parts of your body, which is why it is considered less dangerous than the other two skin cancers that can spread. But even though it does not spread to other parts of your body, the cancer can get worse if not taken care of quickly.

Basal cell lesions can be treated either topically or surgically, both of which have very high rates of success. Efudex, a 5-fluorouracil cream (which is a chemotherapy agent used to treat other cancers), is applied daily to the lesions. The one downside to this monthlong treatment is that the affected area can ooze or weep while the medicine works on the sores. But Efudex offers patients a 91 percent rate of success in getting rid of all cancer cells. This is an ideal treatment for those patients who may not be good candidates for surgery.

If you opt to have the basal cell lesions surgically removed, you can go to either a dermatologist or a plastic surgeon. While most basal cell tumors require only a simple excision, if the lesion is near your eyelid, nose, or lips, please make sure that your doctor uses the Mohs surgical technique. This involves methodically excising the cancerous area one thin slice at a time, examining the excised tissue under a microscope to determine if it contains cancer cells, and continuing the process until the cancer is completely removed. This limits the damage done to the flesh while also making certain that all of the cancer cells have been excised. Mohs surgery offers patients a 99 percent cancer-free success rate. And because the smallest amount of tissue possible has been excised, the chance of a successful reconstructive surgery—if necessary—is greatly increased.

Squamous Cell Carcinoma. Squamous cell lesions often have wartlike features, appearing slightly raised and nodular like a bulb growing partially out of the ground, and can sometimes have layers. You should be aware that squamous cells can develop from noncancerous lesions called actinic keratoses. These red, flat, scaly lesions have a 20 percent chance of turning into squamous cells, so they need to be treated almost as if they were cancer. In other words, you need to take them seriously too.

There is no topical treatment for squamous cell cancer—the tissue must be excised. And because this cancer can spread, it is critical that the surgeon remove *all* cancer cells. Therefore, a larger section of tissue needs to be taken from the area than with basal cell cancer. Because this larger excision can cause some level of disfigurement, a plastic surgeon should perform the procedure.

The noncancerous actinic keratoses, which do not need to be excised, are normally treated topically with a cream called Carac. Carac is a milder version of 5-fluorouracil and has proven to be very successful in removing actinic keratoses as well as other small premalignant lesions.

Malignant Melanoma. This is the most life threatening of the three types of skin cancer. The survival rate is good if the cancer is caught early and the patient receives proper treatment; thus early detection is critical. Malignant melanoma develops at the site of moles on your skin. Of course, most moles are not cancerous, so there is no need to panic just because you have one. The key is to notice any changes to an existing mole and, if you do, have a doctor look at it immediately. In addition, any new mole should be monitored carefully to make sure it does not develop any of the characteristics listed below.

The American Academy of Dermatology has created a handy guide to use for the self-evaluation of moles. I find that my patients easily remember these early warning signs because it follows the progression A-B-C-D.

A is for **asymmetry**. Healthy moles grow out from the center and therefore should appear symmetrical. If one side of a mole looks off center or larger than the other half, you should have it checked.

B is for **border.** Any irregular border or scalloped edge on a mole could be a sign that it is unhealthy. If any mole, new or old, has an uneven border, then you should have your doctor look at it.

C is for **color.** Healthy moles are consistent in color. If a mole exhibits multiple colors (or even different shades of the same color) this could be a sign of trouble. Even if you are not sure, err on the side of caution and have it checked.

D is for **diameter.** A mole is three-dimensional and normally grows up, down, and out. Any mole that becomes larger than the diameter of a pencil eraser should be checked immediately.

Malignant melanoma cancer is directly related to sun exposure, with genetics playing a role as well. Australia has the highest per capita rate of malignant melanoma on earth. Many attribute this to the hole in the ozone layer above that continent, which allows stronger ultraviolet rays into the atmosphere there. Using sunblock is essential to protect yourself. Retin-A has also been shown to reduce the chance of some types of skin cancer (basal and squamous cell) because it is so effective in increasing the turnover time of cells in the epidermis. Yet one more benefit of Retin-A!

FINE LINES AND WRINKLES

Once your dermatologist has determined your skin is healthy, you are free to weigh the many available options for minimizing fine lines and wrinkles. But beware: The skin care industry is awash in hype. It seems every few months a new miracle ingredient, whether it is the bark of a rare tree or the serum of a wild snail, is discovered that will magically erase all of your wrinkles. Perusing some of the ads in fashion magazines I have to wonder why everyone doesn't look 18 years old, since it seems all you have to do is call an 800 number and provide your credit card information. Jokes aside, while there are some very effective products out there, none is truly miraculous.

And the Federal Trade Commission has not helped to dispel the hype. They define fine lines and wrinkles as a lack of moisture. As a result, any product that moisturizes your skin can claim to "reduce fine lines and wrinkles." That doesn't narrow it down much, does it? In order to devise the most effective skin care regimen you need to be able to separate fact from fiction, as well as to understand what best fits into your budget and lifestyle. This chapter will help you do that.

Cosmetic dermatology regimes include the following three categories: at-home maintenance involving creams and cleansers; noninvasive procedures at a doctor's office such as chemical peels; and invasive procedures such as fillers, Botox, and laser treatments.

Since this chapter is about the dermatologist's office, all products I discuss must be acquired through a prescription and all procedures described are performed by a doctor. Even if you are not currently under the care of a dermatologist, however, this chapter offers useful information. At the very least it will give you a point of reference to the ingredients found in over-the-counter products (I'll discuss these products in chapter 4). Keep in mind that the main difference between prescription and nonprescription products is usually one of concentration and degree of activity—the higher the concentration and more effect they have, the more carefully creams and peels need to be applied because of the increased risk of side effects. Therefore, while a prescription-strength retinoid requires a doctor's supervision, it operates in fundamentally the same way as a retinol from your local drugstore, just much more effectively.

Just because you are under the care of a dermatologist does not mean you are immune from hype. Since cosmetic dermatology has become so lucrative, some practitioners have built multimillion-dollar skin care empires that do more for their bottom line than for your skin. Even when visiting your dermatologist you should choose your products carefully—especially since those sold in a doctor's office tend to cost more!

caveat emptor

AT-HOME MAINTENANCE

There are many great products that you can incorporate into your daily skin care regime. The following is a guide to the active ingredients you should look for and what each can offer, either alone or in various combinations.

RETINOIDS

Vitamin A derivatives, retinoids were first used as a topical acne medication. Now they have become an important cornerstone of skin care. Retinoids work in several ways.

First, they exfoliate the stratum corneum, giving your skin a smoother texture. Second, retinoids help disperse the melanocytes of the basal layer more evenly. This results in the elimination of freckles, uneven skin tone, and unsightly blotches. Retinoids also stimulate the fibroblasts in the dermis layer, increasing the production of collagen and elastin. Finally, retinoids inhibit the gene that produces the matrix metalloproteinase enzymes. These enzymes break down collagen and elastin, so anything that inhibits their activity is a good thing. And, if all of the above were not enough, recent studies show that the use of retinoids can actually reduce your risk of skin cancer.

Retinoids come in two forms—creams and gels. Renova, a cream, is great for people with dry skin because it also works as a moisturizer, while Retin-A, a gel, is appropriate for people with normal to oily skin. Since both are offered in varying degrees of concentration and retinoids can irritate the skin, I always suggest that patients start at a lower concentration, working their way up to the lowest possible level that is effective for them. This is important because if a skin irritation does develop, patients may stop using the retinoid before reaping the benefits, making the whole process an exercise in futility. So determining the right formula is not just an issue of comfort; it ensures continued use and positive results.

Retinoids can make your skin more sensitive to the sun, so they should be applied in the evening, just before bedtime. If you do go into the sun the following day you must wear a good sunscreen to limit any irritation. For long-term use, you can only

caveat emptor Over-the-counter retinols come in concentrations so low that it is hard for them to produce visible results. Not only are they too dilute to do much good, nonprescription retinols are not designed to penetrate the skin and treat the fibroblasts like retinoids do, further weakening their overall effectiveness.

SKIN BLEACHES

If discoloration or uneven skin tone is a problem, prescription-strength skin bleach creams can help. The best active ingredient to look for is hydroquinone. The results are usually slow to appear, requiring a long-term commitment, but bleach creams can eventually work. Although thorough studies in the United States have not shown any evidence of increased risk of cancer from using hydroquinone, some European studies have shown a link, so you should speak to your doctor about this concern. For people with significant skin pigmentation problems, a cream called Tri-Luma combines hydroquinone, retinoic acid, and hydrocortisone into a single cream. This product uses the hydroquinone to decrease melanin production, the retinoic acid to disperse melanin granules more evenly, and the hydrocortisone to reduce the inflammation caused by the first two medications.

NONINVASIVE PROCEDURES

Most noninvasive procedures done in a dermatologist's office can be classified as some variety of chemical peel. All peels—even those mini-peels offered by spas—are acid-based. The results of a peel will depend on the active ingredient and the concentration of that ingredient. When deciding which peel is best for you, remember that you usually get what you pay for. A "lunch-hour" peel, for example, will help exfoliate some of the dead skin of the epidermis, but the short downtime should be a clear indication that the acid is not penetrating deeply enough to provide any lasting or noticeable results. The downtime associated with various chemical peels is related to the degree of acidity. The stronger the acidity of a peel, the deeper the layers of skin destruction will be. A lunch-hour peel will be a very superficial peel that leaves a little redness after the treatment. In contrast, deeper peels can require weeks of recovery but with much better improvements in skin texture.

When considering any peel, you must first be aware of the sensitivity of your skin. Those with sensitive skin will not only have increased discomfort during the procedure, but will also take longer to recover after the peel. Because peels are acid-based, they work in the same way as the AHA creams: by traumatizing the skin just enough, the dermal layer reacts by producing more collagen in an effort to protect itself. This trauma results in thicker, more youthful-looking skin. The burning function of a peel obviously exfoliates as well, stripping away the dead, dull skin of the epidermis.

In order to maximize the benefits of a peel, doctors will usually prescribe either a retinoid or an AHA cream to support the collagen production initiated by the peel. The following peels are arranged in order from the weakest to the strongest acid. Expect better results, but longer downtimes, as you move down the list of options.

AHA PEEL

The most common type of peel, an AHA peel usually contains either lactic acid or glycolic acid. The acid concentration can go up to 70 percent, but the formula your practitioner uses on your skin will be determined by its sensitivity. If you are having a peel for the first time, it is always a good idea to be tested behind your ear for 10 minutes before proceeding. Depending on your skin type and the acid concentration, downtimes can vary from a day or two to a week. This peel can be performed four to six times a year. Moisturizing after an AHA peel is important, as is applying either a retinoid or an AHA cream.

JESSNER'S PEEL

This acid peel is very high in strength but can still be done without anesthesia. Keep in mind that the Jessner's peel is much stronger than even the most highly concentrated AHA peel, so your skin will be upset for at least five days. Of course, longer downtimes usually represent better results, which is the case with the Jessner's peel. People with sensitive skin should proceed with extreme caution when considering a Jessner's peel because there can be a significant sensation of burning during the procedure. If skin sensitivity is not an issue, the Jessner's peel offers a good balance between impressive results and a low risk of any serious burning or scars.

TCA PEEL

This peel is extremely effective but does straddle the pain threshold and thus may require local anesthesia. The active ingredient, trichloroacetic acid, is offered in varying concentrations. (Any TCA peel with a concentration of 35 percent or higher must be performed while under anesthesia.) Because a TCA peel is so effective in getting rid of fine lines and wrinkles it is very often done in conjunction with a facelift. A TCA peel can be performed around the mouth at the same time as the facial surgery, but in any other area of the face you must wait at least three months after a facelift before having the peel. Due to their strength, TCA peels should only be performed about once a year. The one main downside to such a strong peel is that if it is not mixed properly or if the dosage is off, the acid can damage your skin, possibly even leaving scars. So considering a TCA peel is serious business and you should only go to a doctor who does them often. The Obagi Blue Peel, a milder version of a regular TCA peel, offers a shorter downtime, but, as one would guess, less improvement than a 35 percent TCA peel. You should discuss the pros and cons of each with your doctor before deciding which one is right for you.

PHENOL PEEL

Strongest of all, the phenol peel—whose active ingredient is phenolic acid—is the most effective in reducing fine lines and wrinkles. In my experience, these rather dramatic results are unmatched by any other type of skin treatment. However, the one downside—and it should be considered carefully—is that it causes severe hypopigmentation in almost all patients. Hypopigmentation causes the skin to turn pale white, thus this peel is absolutely not an option for anyone with a darker complexion. Because of its strength, a phenol peel is only performed when the patient is under anesthesia. And, like a TCA peel, this peel is often done in conjunction with a facelift, with the same dictates regarding areas of the face and timing as the TCA peel. Studies have shown that a phenol peel can cause heart arrhythmias both during and after the procedure, especially in people who have existing heart and liver problems. Therefore, this peel should only be performed on healthy people in a medically supervised environment.

INVASIVE PROCEDURES

Beyond the various peels, there are other procedures your dermatologist can perform to help with fine lines and wrinkles. These include muscle-paralyzing agents (Botox), fillers (temporary and permanent), and laser treatments. Since Botox, fillers, and lasers operate in the deep layers of your skin these procedures are considered more invasive and should be approached with a degree of caution. The results are usually more pronounced, but the risk of a less-than-perfect outcome is also higher. The fact that they tend to cost considerably more than noninvasive procedures should help you take them more seriously.

There is a troubling trend in recent years of many of these treatments being performed by untrained technicians. Beware of a spa offering Botox or laser treatments at a steep discount—this is probably an indication that a properly trained doctor will not be performing your procedure. Believe it or not, this area is not as regulated as it should be and laws as to who can wield a laser, for example, vary from state to state. A good rule of thumb is to never let anyone but a well-trained doctor—either a board-certified plastic surgeon or dermatologist—do any of these procedures.

MUSCLE-PARALYZING AGENTS (BOTOX)

Botox injections have become the most commonly performed aesthetic procedure in the United States. Botox, a protein produced by the bacterium *Clostridium botulinum*, has the ability to paralyze muscles. Doctors inject very small amounts to areas of the face where muscles cause wrinkles, so that once the targeted muscle has been paralyzed, the wrinkles simply disappear. Although people may have shuddered initially at the idea of deliberately inducing paralysis of facial muscles, no matter how slight, Botox has been tested for more than 30 years and is now considered completely safe when performed in a controlled environment. Recently, the FDA has approved a new form of Botulinum Toxin called Dysport. This drug will be very similar to Botox, except some early reviews suggest that it may last longer, have an earlier onset of action, and be less expensive.

The most common area to be injected is between your eyebrows, as this is the muscle responsible for those unattractive furrows on your forehead. Not only is Botox a great way to nonsurgically smooth out wrinkles, but its resounding success is also based on the fact that Botox requires little or no downtime, which is quite extraordinary considering the results. The typical Botox injection lasts from three to six months, depending on the concentration of the formula and the size of the muscle being treated. Because men usually have larger muscles—even in their faces—they require more Botox per treatment, or they can expect a shorter-acting result. On the downside, if Botox migrates toward the muscles of the upper eyelid it can cause temporary sagging in that area. Although this condition can be reversed with medication, it is certainly not the result a Botox patient is looking for!

In addition to removing wrinkles, Botox can be used to reduce sweating in those who perspire excessively, to treat muscle tension headaches, and for nonsurgical brow lifts (see chapter 7).

The following is a list of muscles that can be treated with Botox.

Facial Muscle	Anatomical Area	Effect of Botox Treatment
corrugator supercilli	between eyebrows (vertical lines)	eliminates frown lines
procerus	between eyebrows (horizontal lines)	eliminates horizontal lines on bridge of the nose
frontalis	forehead (horizontal lines)	eliminates forehead lines, lifts corner of eyebrow
orbicularis oculi	corner of eye (crow's-feet)	relaxes crow's-feet, lifts corner of eyebrow
orbicularis oris	vertical lines around the mouth	softens lines around the mouth
mentalis	dimpling on the chin	relaxes dimpling on the chin
platysma	vertical bands on the neck	relaxes vertical bands
nasalis	wrinkling on the side of the nose when smiling	softens wrinkling on the side of the nose

FILLERS

While Botox smoothes out your skin by manipulating the underlying cause of the wrinkles (the muscle), fillers work in a different way by repairing the actual injury to the skin. Fillers are very effective in correcting soft tissue loss and repairing any changes to the contours of your face due to sagging tissue, weight loss, or acne. Deep wrinkles such as those around your mouth and nose (nasolabial folds, marionette lines, tear trough depressions) as well as the furrows on your forehead respond well to the use of fillers. While some physicians will inject fillers in the crow's-feet area, I do not. The skin in this area is very thin and I feel there is a risk of actually seeing the filler underneath. Also, the muscle causing the wrinkles is strong and can push the filler around, creating even deeper grooves—the exact opposite of the desired result! Therefore, I avoid placing filler in that area and treat those wrinkles with Botox instead.

Temporary Fillers. As the name suggests, temporary fillers will dissolve over time. I like temporary fillers because your face changes as you age and these will not disrupt the natural shifts of soft tissue as permanent fillers can. The important thing with any temporary filler is to make sure your doctor is experienced enough to inject it in the proper places. If not, the end result can look bumpy and somewhat unnatural. There are four types of temporary synthetic fillers.

Collagen. Most often derived from the skin of a cow, collagen is the least expensive temporary filler. There is a 3 percent chance of an adverse reaction to the bovine collagen, so a small test is usually performed first. Injected collagen lasts about three months and costs $400 per milliliter. There are new synthetically derived or cadaveric human collagens available that will not cause allergic reactions. However, the cost is significantly higher than bovine collagen and the filler still only lasts about three months.

Hyaluronic Acid (HA). Marketed under the names Restylane, Juvéderm, Hyalaform, and Captique, hyaluronic acid is the favored temporary filler option of most doctors. Hyaluronic acid is a repeating chain of sugar molecules that retains water, thus plumping up the skin. Because your body is constantly breaking down its own HA, these fillers have been specifically formulated with cross-linking capability to resist this rapid breakdown. Therefore, depending on the brand, HA can last anywhere from 6 to 12 months. All HAs are easily injected and do not require a reactivity test because there is no known allergic reaction to it. Hyaluronic acid costs from $600 to $1,000 per milliliter.

Calcium Hydroxyapatite Crystals. Marketed under the name Radiesse, this filler consists of ground-up bone granules. The bones used are not harvested from cadavers (despite a persistent urban legend to the contrary); rather, they are manufactured through a chemical process. Radiesse is best used in areas requiring large amounts of filler because the granules are big. Conversely, their size makes them inappropriate for filling finer wrinkles. This filler is more painful to inject than other types of temporary fillers and, as such, requires a regional or local anesthesia to make it more tolerable. Also, this filler should not be used in the lips because of the risk of severe bumpiness. The cost is from $1,000 to $1,500 per 1.3 cc (which is slightly more than a milliliter). While the cost per cc is approximately the same as for hyaluronic acid, these fillers can last up to 24 months, which does make them more cost effective.

Poly-L-lactic Acid. Known as Sculptra, poly-L-lactic acid is a temporary filler that is currently only available to HIV patients who are looking to correct the loss of soft tissue in their face (facial lipoatrophy). Sculptra, when injected, creates a temporary inflammation that eventually adds more volume to the skin tissue by increasing collagen production. The problem is that, because the results from each session can take up to two months to present themselves, it is difficult for doctors to determine the precise amount of fill that has been generated during each session. As a result, accuracy can be compromised. Also, the process is a bit demanding because it requires multiple injections over the course of an extended period of time before seeing noticeable results. Finally, since the increased volume is the result of inflammation, some patients can end up looking severely swollen or bumpy.

Fat. While there are several nonsynthetic fillers from which to choose (fat, fascia, dermis), your own fat is now considered the best option for a variety of reasons. Fat is your own tissue and thus poses no threat of an allergic reaction. Fat is also easy to harvest (most of us have a virtually unlimited supply) with minimal pain, and the procedure leaves no visible scarring. Finally, I consider fat's strongest selling point is that it is inexpensive. Other fillers are extremely cost prohibitive, especially when working in areas that require large amounts. When a doctor harvests fat from a patient the cost is the same whether 1 cc or 10 cc is taken out. Using fat as a filler has also become easier because of technological advances made in the way it is harvested. In the past, fat was thought to "melt away" from the injection site and for that reasons was not the primary choice of doctors. However, newer techniques now minimize cell damage while maximizing the extraction of viable tissue. The Viafill system has been designed to increase the number of live fat cells that are injected, thus increasing the long-term durability of fat injections. Because of all these reasons, fat has now become the filler of choice for cheek and chin augmentation, lip enlargement, and correcting nasolabial folds, marionette lines, and overall facial volume loss.

Location	Choice of Fillers	Best Treatment
forehead wrinkles	hyaluronic acid, calcium hydroxyapatite	Botox
frown lines	hyaluronic acid	Botox, followed by hyaluronic acid
crow's-feet	hyaluronic acid	Botox only
nasal deformities	calcium hydroxyapatite	calcium hydroxyapatite
tear trough deformities	fat, hyaluronic acid, calcium hydroxyapatite	fat
nasolabial folds	fat, hyaluronic acid, calcium hydroxyapatite	fine lines: hyaluronic acid; deeper folds: fat or calcium hydroxyapatite
marionette lines	fat, hyaluronic acid, calcium hydroxyapatite	fine lines: hyaluronic acid; deeper folds: fat or calcium hydroxyapatite
lip plumping	fat, hyaluronic acid	fat
smoker's lines on lips	hyaluronic acid	hyaluronic acid
volume replacement, cheek and chin augmentation	fat, calcium hydroxyapatite, Sculptra	fat

Permanent Fillers. I do not use permanent fillers because they are permanent. I have seen plenty of patients whose 10-year-old injections end up looking out of place on their face. When your facial anatomy changes and soft tissue starts to sag, what seemed like the right spot for a filler can very easily turn into the wrong spot. The most important thing to remember about a permanent filler is that once it is injected into your face it is going to stay there—so you better like it! (And you better like it in 20 years, too.) Temporary fillers accomplish the same results but with more forgiveness, so I see no reason to incur the risks attached to permanent fillers.

Although I do not recommend using permanent fillers, there are two types currently being offered in the marketplace: silicone beads and silicone droplets.

Silicone Beads. Sold under the brand name Artecoll, these tiny round balls of silicone (the size of red blood cells) are injected into the dermis. Beyond the fact that Artecoll is permanent, I have additional concerns. First, there is some bovine collagen in the mixture, so there could be an allergic reaction to it. Second, and more worrying, is that if the Artecoll is not injected properly it can lead to inflammation. This can cause permanent scarring under the skin, which presents itself in the form of a bumpy texture that is visible to the naked eye even though the scarring has occurred at the dermal layer.

Silicone Droplets. A type of silicone that has been formulated into microdroplets is injected into your dermis, which causes the fibroblasts to form new collagen around these droplets. As the new collagen is produced it fills in the wrinkles of the targeted area. Again, while the initial results may be good, this filler is being placed in the soft tissue of your face and can never be moved or removed. There is also the risk of inflammation and scarring both from the injection and from the resulting growth of collagen around the droplets.

Final warning: Stay away from silicone and any other permanent fillers!

LASER TREATMENTS

As with my disclosure regarding permanent fillers, I will state upfront that I do not advise the use of laser treatments as a rejuvenating tool. I think peels offer the same benefits without the risks. But since they are being offered in the marketplace you should understand what they do and why I object to their use.

Laser treatment for fine lines and wrinkles came onto the dermatological scene in the 1990s. Previously, the only available treatments for these problems were deep chemical peels and dermabrasion. Chemical peels, which are generally considered very effective in treating fine lines and wrinkles, can sometimes be problematic because of inconsistencies in pH and concentration levels. And dermabrasion, while an excellent technique for getting rid of fine lines and wrinkles, requires a surgical skill that many dermatologists and plastic surgeons do not have. Because of these occasional problems with peels and dermabrasion, the first laser (the CO_2 laser) was welcomed onto the dermatological scene with much fanfare. Yet since the very beginning doctors have recognized certain limitations to laser treatments. As a result, every few years a "new and improved" machine is introduced that offers different technology. Not even the newer machines have convinced me this is a good way to get rid of fine lines and wrinkles when viable alternatives exist.

Aside from facial rejuvenation, lasers have many other compelling reasons for their use. They are excellent at removing tattoos or other colored blemishes on your skin. They are good for removal of unwanted blood vessels, as well as unwanted hair. But fine lines and wrinkles are still better treated with other methods.

Lasers work in different ways, and the best laser treatment for you depends on what problem you are trying to correct. Here is a brief overview of the various categories:

Laser Absorbed By	Good For
red pigments	correction of broken blood vessels, unwanted redness of the skin, removal of tattoos with red/orange pigments
brown pigments	pigmentary problems, brown spots, black/brown tattoo removal
water	exfoliation, dermal injury repair, skin resurfacing
the pigment in the hair follicle	permanent hair removal

The following different types of laser machines are currently being used by dermatologists.

CO_2 Laser. The first laser designed to treat skin problems, the CO_2 laser basically performs the same functions as a TCA peel or dermabrasion. It helps get rid of dead skin, evens out skin tone, and smooths fine lines and wrinkles. The CO_2 laser also stimulates the fibroblasts in the dermis to make more collagen while at the same time contracting existing collagen fibrils—both resulting in tighter-looking skin. Immediately following a

CO_2 laser treatment a patient will have raw, red, weeping skin and will probably develop scabs in the areas that have been treated. CO_2 lasers are less complex than today's hybrids in that their light energy is evenly distributed across the top of the skin, thus causing injury to the entire skin surface. Treatments from a CO_2 laser can result in severe hypopigmentation, much like a phenol peel. The downtime for this laser treatment can be as much as six weeks, much longer than most peels. Results tend to last one to two years.

Erbium Laser. This machine was introduced in an effort to achieve some of the same things the CO_2 laser could do, but without the side effects. It works by using a laser light energy that does not heat up the skin to the same degree as the CO_2 laser does. While an erbium laser offers a shortened recovery time and little risk of hypopigmentation, the results are mild to minimal, so it is hard to justify the expense and inconvenience of the treatment.

Nonablative Laser. The next generation of laser technology uses limited energy to heat up the skin in order to stimulate the fibroblasts into making more collagen while not injuring the epidermis. I find these nonablative lasers the least impressive of all laser techniques. The results are minimal, offering less marked changes than even the erbium laser. And the cost is prohibitive (which has much to do with the physician attempting to recoup the hefty purchase price of the machine). To show any noticeable improvement patients must often undergo 10 to 15 treatments—you can do the math! All of this might be acceptable if the nonablative laser were the only option— but it isn't. You would be much better off having any type of peel done.

Fraxel Laser. These most recent lasers, available in CO_2 or erbium varieties, are by far the best, although I still do not think either offers better results than a peel. The idea behind the Fraxel lasers is to reduce the amount of injury to the skin. So while the CO_2 laser would go across the entire surface, these new lasers offer a sort of "polka dot" treatment, with the majority of the skin remaining untouched by the laser. Although only small areas of skin are worked on, wrinkles do disappear across the entire face since the fibroblasts have been stimulated to produce more collagen. This result is achieved without causing severe hypopigmentation or a long postoperative recovery time. Overall, while Fraxel lasers are the best laser treatments currently in the marketplace, I am still not convinced that they provide patients with any advantage over a peel, and they cost much more.

OTHER DERMATOLOGICAL CONCERNS

Laser	Uses	Limitations	# of Treatments
pulsed dye laser	facial redness, scars, fine blood vessels, broken capillaries	mild redness and swelling for 1–2 days	3–4
Q-switched Nd:YAG	brown spots, dark-colored tattoos	very subtle results	4–10
intense pulsed light (IPL)	photo facials, hair removal, brown/red blemish removal	"jack of all trades, master of none," highest rate of burns and hypopigmentation	3–4
Thermage	skin tightening, wrinkle reduction	radiofrequency (not a laser), no convincing results	1–2
Fraxel erbium	skin discoloration, fine wrinkles, photo-damage, acne scars	2–3 days of redness	3–4
Fraxel CO_2		10 days of crusting and redness	
Portrait (nitrogen plasma)	nonlaser device for fine lines and wrinkles	painful, 7–14 day downtime with crusting	1–2
Isolaze (combination vacuum plus IPL)	acne	modest improvement, may be too expensive for the degree of improvement	monthly

Aside from the routine concerns of fine lines, wrinkles, and suspicious moles, dermatologists also have to deal with issues related to the blood vessels under the skin. Below I describe the basic treatments for these maladies as well as assorted dermatologic treatments, including tattoo removal, laser hair removal, and pigment changes.

VARICOSE VEINS, BROKEN BLOOD VESSELS, AND CAPILLARIES

If you have any noticeable red, blue, or purple blood vessels on your body or face, a dermatologist can offer two types of treatments to get rid of them. A pulsed dye laser can burn them away while an injectable solution can dissolve them. If the problem area is on your face, you should only consider a laser treatment, as the injectable solution is unsafe to use that close to your brain. Laser treatments work by directing a pinpointed light energy to the blood vessels, heating them up and causing them to coagulate. This coagulated substance is then absorbed by your body, thereby making the discoloration disappear.

Sclerotherapy uses a microneedle to inject a substance into broken blood vessels at intervals of approximately 1 inch (2 to 3 cm). The injected sclerosing agent causes the vessel to clot and eventually disappear. Because the sclerosing solution is mild and the needles so small, there is not a lot of discomfort associated with this procedure, even when it involves multiple injections, which it usually does. A minimum of two or more sessions is often necessary to ensure the vein will no longer be visible.

TATTOO REMOVAL

Laser technology can now safely and successfully remove that permanent tattoo you have regretted for years, without even leaving a scar. It is not a quick or an easy process, but it can be done. A laser is directed at the ink of the tattoo, the light is absorbed into the skin, the ink is broken up into small fragments, and then those fragments are naturally cleansed out of your system. Different lasers treat different color inks, based on their varying wavelengths, so the removal of a multicolored tattoo will require more sessions than a monochromatic one. It will typically take two or three laser treatments to adequately remove a professional multicolored tattoo. Be aware that when lasers remove tattoo pigment they also remove the natural pigments in your skin, so the final result can often have a hypopigmented look. Amateur tattoos are more difficult to remove completely, as they are often embedded into different skin layers.

Overall, laser tattoo removal is probably the safest way to go, as it is the least invasive. Most patients consider the process relatively painless, although there can be a slight burning sensation after each treatment. The number of sessions needed will depend on the color, size, and depth of your tattoo. If you require multiple treatments they should be performed at least five weeks apart in order to accurately show the full effects of the previous treatment (the ink needs time to flush out of your body). There can also be some swelling and redness after each session, so it is a good idea to rest the area before another treatment.

LASER HAIR REMOVAL

There are many different lasers that can help permanently remove unwanted hair. The biggest advantage of laser hair removal versus electrolysis is that lasers can treat a much larger area in a considerably shorter period of time. Electrolysis is labor-intensive, requiring hair to be removed one follicle at a time, so it can take months to achieve the desired results. The two best lasers for hair removal are the Diode laser and the Alexandrite laser. For dark-skinned patients, the laser of choice is the long-pulsed Nd:YAG.

SKIN PIGMENT CHANGES

There are three ways that dermatologists can treat skin pigment issues: chemical peels, laser treatments, and Tri-Luma, a topical treatment. I would avoid using a laser to remove unwanted pigmentation because it can cause hypopigmentation in the area, making it look worse than before the treatment. Both chemical peels and topical treatments can produce strong results. Chemical peels are especially effective in dispersing the melanin granules of the epidermis that are causing the uneven skin tone. But, of course, they do require a certain amount of downtime that might be difficult to accommodate. If this is the case, the cream Tri-Luma is very effective. Consisting of Retin-A, hydroquinone, and cortisone (which is added to reduce the irritation caused by the Retin-A), Tri-Luma will gradually disperse the melanin granules that are responsible for the discoloration.

HOW MUCH WILL IT COST?

Treatment	Cost per Treatment[†]	Frequency
chemical peels	$250–750	depending on the type of peel, 1–6 per year
Botox	$400–1,200 (depending on how much Botox is used)	every 3–6 months
collagen	$400–600	every 3 months
hyaluronic acid	$650–800	every 6–12 months
Radiesse	$800–1,200	every 12–24 months
fat injections	$1,200–2,500	every 12–48 months
laser treatments	$600–1,500	varies with type of laser
sclerotherapy	$250–500	2 treatments per area

[†]Note: All prices are in U.S. dollars, current as of 2009.

Internet Resources: Dermatology and Skin

www.aad.org/public/index.html

Internet Resources: Facial Fillers and Botox

www.injectablesafety.org

Chapter 4

BEAUTY IN A BOTTLE

"When you have two pennies left in the world, buy a loaf of bread with one, and a lily with the other."

—Chinese Proverb

Despite the constant bombardment of advertising and marketing campaigns that promise otherwise, most skin care products sold without a prescription are little more than glorified moisturizers. And that is equally true of a $4 bottle of cream at Walgreens as it is of a $400 jar of seaweed-infused serum at Bergdorf Goodman. Of course, hydration adds to the overall health of your skin, so a good moisturizer is an important part of any comprehensive skin care regime. But all of the fancy packaging and incredible claims are designed to perpetrate the enduring myth that these products can somehow transform the way you look. They can't.

Nevertheless, at one point or another you will have to negotiate the aisles of CVS. Whether you are under the care of a dermatologist and need supplemental products or are relying on over-the-counter products as your sole means of skin care, it helps to understand what you can (and cannot) expect from them. By unraveling the hype that surrounds this multibillion-dollar industry, you will acquire the tools necessary to choose products that are right for you. And after reading this chapter I am quite sure your shopping list will not only be shorter but the products will also cost less.

SEPARATING FACT FROM FICTION

There is not a huge amount of regulatory oversight in the area of over-the-counter skin care products. This, in itself, is a good indication that these products are not particularly strong. Two U.S. governmental agencies—the Food and Drug Administration (FDA) and the Federal Trade Commission (FTC)—are responsible for monitoring the industry. The FDA's main requirement is that manufacturers must list the complete ingredients on the package and must not promise consumers a permanent result. The FTC, which is more concerned with truth-in-advertising issues, regulates claims made about what a product can do.

Because oversight standards are so lax, cosmetics companies have found easy ways to sell their products without breaking the rules. By using phrases like "seems to," "appears to," "you may experience," and "feels as if" when describing their products, they are not making any actual guarantees even as they strongly suggest the product is worth your hard-earned dollars.

Another marketing trick (and it is a trick) is to use phrases like "laboratory tested" or "studies show" to help sell a product. If a manufacturer pays an independent lab to conduct tests that are sure to favor their product, they are not breaking any FTC rule if they then use these skewed results in promoting the product. Serious scientific inquiry demands *peer-reviewed* studies, which are rarely—if ever—the type financed by cosmetics or skin care companies. Simply mentioning a test does not mean the results can be trusted. Was the study controlled? How many people were tested? Who paid for the test? A critical look at these studies would no doubt reveal that they have been done for one reason only—to help market, advertise, and sell a product. All of which does not add up to very sound science.

When sifting through the hype, you should also look for certain catchphrases that are designed to sound important but mean nothing in terms of the actual chemistry of the product. Terms like "hypoallergenic," "noncomedogenic," and "designed for sensitive skin" are not regulated by the FDA or FTC, so they can mean anything the manufacturer wants them to mean. For example, certain ingredients may be more allergenic than others, but none causes a reaction in everyone. So which ingredients have been left out in order to call a product hypoallergenic? More than likely, some marketing guru has told the New Products Division that consumers are worried about allergens this year and—presto—the company introduces a "hypoallergenic" line. I should point out that, unlike more serious misrepresentations I cover in other chapters, none of these hyped-up marketing ploys of over-the-counter products will actually hurt you. Rather, they are just annoying distractions that are designed to separate you from your money.

Celebrity endorsements and customer testimonials are another marketing tool that does not add up to much in the way of product information. Just because a beautiful 20-year-old actress uses a face cream (and who knows if she actually does use it) in no way means that your skin will look like hers. And why should a naturally attractive person—who did not achieve her beauty but rather was born with it—suddenly become an expert on the subject of skin care? Complicating the situation are questions that usually remain unanswered when it comes to celebrity spokespeople: Was she paid an endorsement fee? Does she own part of the company? Or does she really just like the product? These same questions apply to "everyday people" testimonials that are often used to hawk the most suspect of skin care products. Unfortunately these types of sales pitches are used over and over again because they work! Just remember that as long as the ingredients are listed on the package and the manufacturer does not promise permanent results these ads can say just about anything, and they usually do.

Finally, the old adage "you get what you pay for" does not necessarily apply to over-the-counter skin care products. I am always amazed at what people are willing to spend based solely on slick packaging, suspect claims, and exotic-sounding ingredients that add nothing to the overall effectiveness of a product. Once you start paying attention to ingredient lists you will see that there is little variation across the broad spectrum of price points. In fact, some larger conglomerates that own a number of skin care companies sell the same formulas under different product names and at *very* different prices. It seems that when it comes to skin care products people trust blindly in the notion that high cost equals high quality—and that is very often not the case.

Although people are eager to believe in an easy fix, the reality is that if any single ingredient were discovered that made everyone look years younger, we would all be using it. Instead, the market is flooded with thousands of products that all claim to offer you the fountain of youth. The bottom line is that these products are basically just moisturizers. So my advice is to ignore the hype of dermatologist-tested, celebrity-endorsed expensive creams and just find the products that work best on your skin. You will probably save plenty of money doing so.

COSMECEUTICALS

As the name implies, this group of hybrid products combines pharmaceutical ingredients with cosmetics. However, because the concentration of the pharmaceuticals is low, they do not require a prescription, thus widening the potential market for these products. The production and marketing of cosmeceuticals has become big business. These products are usually more expensive than your standard skin care products and all of them promise improved results. But just because they cost more and are being promoted by an authoritative doctor wearing a white coat doesn't necessarily mean they work.

As was pointed out in the previous chapter, pharmaceuticals such as retinoids and alpha hydroxy acids improve the condition of your skin by affecting the biological processes of your soft tissue. The scientific fact is that a retinol found in a cosmeceutical is not going to make the same improvements that a retinoid will make. Nor will an alpha hydroxy acid with a high pH offer the same results as one with a lower, more acidic, pH. No matter what the cosmeceutical ad campaigns promise, the science simply does not support their claims because the pharmaceutical ingredients are not as bioactive at that concentration. In the end, cosmeceutical products generally offer more than a simple moisturizer but far less than prescription-strength results.

So why even manufacture them? Part of the answer lies in the fact that doctors make no money when they write prescriptions but can earn a profit when they sell a product. I admit that sounds cynical, but I find it hard not to be when it comes to cosmeceuticals. While it is understandable that cosmetic and skin care companies overhype their latest product, I find it off-putting when a doctor (who understands the basic science of skin care) does the same. These doctors have become no more than salespeople in a perfect position to exploit the situation to their benefit because of their supposed expertise. Their motives seem to be more about ego and money rather than honestly trying to improve the lives of patients.

Another overhyped type of product is the doctor's own label product. With few exceptions, most physicians do not invent or devise their own cosmeceutical lines. These products are devised by outside laboratories and then assembled for a fee with the physician's own labels and packaging. So what is the doctor really selling? Just more of the same overhyped fancy moisturizing creams. Of course there are a few true scientists in the field who truly create their own products; unfortunately for them, the rest of the physicians have spoiled their credibility as pioneers.

Beyond the "doctor-in-a-white-coat" hype, cosmeceuticals seem especially prone to bogus studies, celebrity endorsements, and exaggerated claims. Remember that, unlike pharmaceuticals, these products are barely regulated. Other than requiring that they list ingredients and not promise permanent improvements, the FDA and FTC have little control over this growing industry. So my advice regarding cosmeceuticals is that if you are willing to spend the extra money on these products, recognize that you are not getting much more than glorified moisturizers that have been wrapped up in fancy packaging.

THE "ALL NATURAL" FALLACY

Just because a cosmetic or face cream promotes itself as "natural" does not necessarily mean it is better. In fact, there are quite a number of natural ingredients that can cause allergic reactions, irritate the skin, and lead to dermatitis. In addition, some botanicals can spoil and grow bacteria (just like food) and require artificial preservatives to prolong their shelf life—defeating the whole purpose of being "natural"! A perfect example of this is a spoil-proof form of coconut oil, sodium coco sulfate. The sulfate in that formula comes from sulfuric acid, which should seem a bit out of place in a product being promoted as "botanical" or "natural."

These terms are often used to imply safety, yet natural or botanical products are no more regulated that the rest of the skin care industry. And the irony is that, unlike the benign (if overhyped) claims of synthetic products, more than a few natural or botanical ingredients can actually *cause* skin problems. Some of the more irritating ingredients include almond extract, basil, balsam, citrus, lavender oil, papaya, peppermint, sage, rose, witch hazel, and wintergreen. Of course, any adverse reaction would depend on the concentration of the ingredient and the person's skin. But my point is that just because an ingredient is natural does not necessarily make it safe for everyone. Arsenic is natural, too, but it can kill you. I am not suggesting botanical or natural skin care products can kill you, only that they are not as inherently safe as their marketing campaigns would have you believe.

Truly soothing botanicals such as aloe vera, green tea, kola extract, and licorice root are worth looking for in any list of ingredients. But keep in mind that even though synthetic ingredients, like silicone, are hard to glamorize, it does not mean they do not do a great job moisturizing your skin (silicone does). Further, some of the old-fashioned ingredients that we are led to assume do not measure up to the natural ones, like mineral oil and petroleum jelly, *are* natural (although not botanical). Once again, marketing hype trumps scientific truth, with the net result being that consumers pay more for products that deliver less while the manufacturers laugh all the way to the bank.

This is not to say that all botanical or natural products are bad for you or that they cannot be good for you. I am only advising that you should not assume they are automatically better than a synthetic product, because sometimes they are not. Learn to sift through the hype, read the list of ingredients carefully, and then buy the product with which you are most comfortable.

DAILY SKIN CARE USING OVER-THE-COUNTER PRODUCTS

Comprehensive at-home skin care includes three steps: cleansing, exfoliating, and moisturizing. Most skin care companies want you to buy into the idea that it is much more complicated that that, requiring a cabinet full of products to achieve healthy-looking skin. But since the main goal of any skin care company is to make as much money as possible, it follows that they are going to try to sell you whatever they can, even if it is something you do not need. I cannot blame them for trying, but I can help you separate fact from fiction, saving you money along the way.

CLEANSERS

While this may come as a surprise, a mild cleanser is appropriate for all skin types. Liquid cleansers tend to be milder than bars of soap because the solidifiers that hold a bar together are slightly caustic (that applies to Dove, too). Mild liquid cleansers should be used on acne-prone skin as well because caustic cleansers can inflame the skin, which actually causes the production of more oil. And since most acne (although not all) is caused by hormonal problems found below the skin level, no cleanser is going to clear the acne up anyway. A good, all-purpose mild cleanser that can be used by everyone is Cetaphil, which is found in the skin care aisle of most pharmacies and supermarkets.

EXFOLIANTS

There are a number of nonpharmaceutical exfoliating products on the market that work quite well in sloughing off the dead skin of the epidermis. Exfoliators can either be mechanical, like a Buf-Puf or washcloth, or they can come in the form of facial scrubs that contain a granular substance, either natural or synthetic. How often you exfoliate really depends on the thickness of your skin but, generally speaking, once a week is a good goal to shoot for. Just remember that too much of a good thing can be bad, so do not overdo it. Keep in mind that a callous, that hard, thickened area of skin on your palm or foot, is also caused by too much mechanical irritation. Too much exfoliation will injure the skin and create a leathery appearance.

MOISTURIZERS

This is the area where skin care companies have really got a lucrative racket going. You can now find moisturizers designed exclusively for different types of skin, age groups, and specific areas of your face. Believe me when I say that choosing products based on these niche categories, which were probably invented by the marketing department rather than the research lab, is not going to improve your skin by any measurable amount. Moisture is moisture, and whether it is applied to your eyelid or cheek it is going to have the same positive effect. Any moisturizing ingredient found in a specially designed nighttime cream for the neck is going to be equally effective (or ineffective) on another part of your face. Selecting moisturizers based on skin type is also a bit of a trap in that it does not take into account external environmental factors that can change from season to season. Levels of humidity, dryness, and sun exposure—which greatly affect your skin—vary depending on what time of year it is and where you are, so no one has an absolute fixed skin type. Finally, your age has little to do with choosing the right nonprescription moisturizer because it implies that products designed for older people will be more effective in dealing with the signs of aging—and over-the-counter products are not strong enough to do this. Taking all of this into consideration, my advice regarding moisturizers is to find one that works well for your skin and use it where and when you need it. Period.

SUN PROTECTION

The issue of protecting your skin against the sun is dealt with throughout this book because sun exposure is such a determining factor in how your skin looks. Unprotected sun exposure is also a major cause of skin cancer—which can kill you—so I will not apologize for repeating myself endlessly about how important sunblocks are! And the more you know about which types work (and which do not) the better protected you will be.

Most consumers look to SPF (sun protection factor) of a sunblock as the most important information about that product. Choosing based on SPF alone is a misstep that can have quite detrimental consequences. Thankfully, over-the-counter sunblocks will soon have a more complete sun protection rating system that will provide information on three distinct variables: the SPF as it relates to UVB protection, a four-star rating as it relates to UVA protection, and the sunblock's ability to resist water. Most sunblocks protect against UVB rays—the intense ultraviolet rays of the summer months and peak sunshine hours (10 a.m. to 2 p.m.). While that protection is important, UVA rays are with us 365 days a year, so they should be a serious consideration as well. Therefore, this new rating system will clarify exactly what you are buying and what you will be protecting yourself against.

There are two general types of sunscreens—chemical and physical. A chemical sunscreen absorbs the UV rays while a physical sunscreen reflects the harmful rays away from your skin like a temporary coat of armor. I prefer the physical sunscreens because they block both UVA and UVB rays so you are completely protected throughout the year. Both zinc oxide and titanium dioxide now come in micronized versions that go on as clear creams. Between the two, I advise my patients to use zinc oxide because it offers coverage across the broadest spectrum of UVA rays.

The two most effective ingredients against UVA rays in chemical sunscreens are ecamsule (Mexoryl SX) and avobenzone because they block both UVA and UVB rays. However, because they allow the sun to penetrate your skin, they do not prevent the production of free radicals, which is another reason to favor physical sunblocks. It has also been reported that avobenzone will produce more free radicals as a result of its absorbance of those nasty UVA and UVB rays. Finally, avobenzone breaks down into inactive ingredients within 20 minutes of sun exposure, so in spite of a high SPF rating as a result of other active ingredients in many sunscreens, the most important ingredient may not be beneficial for solar protection in as little as 20 minutes.

If you use chemical sun protection, a strong antioxidant cream (like those found in a doctor's office) should be used in conjunction to counteract the formation of free radicals. Another downside to chemical sunscreens is that they must be applied at least 30 minutes prior to going out in the sun to ensure proper absorption by your skin. While in theory this seems doable, sometimes in the real world it is not. This important requisite is further complicated by the fact that any antioxidant cream needs to be applied first or it won't be absorbed properly, and neither the antioxidant nor the sunblock should be applied over makeup. All of which adds up to the likelihood that one of these steps will be forgotten or not done in time and weaken the overall effectiveness of the chemical sunblock.

No matter which sunblock you choose, there are a few general guidelines to which you should adhere. The product should be water resistant, even if you do not plan to swim, to ensure that you will not perspire it off. Sunscreens should be applied liberally and often regardless of their SPF. Keep in mind that the use of a sunscreen is probably one of the few times when too much of a good thing is a good thing!

ACNE

Although acne is typically associated with the hormonal changes of puberty, people of all ages can suffer from it. Acne is caused by the overproduction of oil that becomes "trapped" in the skin by clogged sebaceous glands located in the dermis. This type of blockage can occur not only because of changes in hormone levels but also because of poor personal hygiene or heavy emotional stress.

The primary focus in fighting acne is usually to decrease oil production. But since over-the-counter products are topical and cannot affect your hormones, they have to approach the problem from a slightly different angle. Just beware that no matter which product you use, overdrying the skin will make the acne worse. Your body will sense the deficiency and actually produce more oil. Therefore, it is important to follow the recommended dosage to ensure optimum results. In other words, doubling the dose will not clear up your acne twice as fast! Beyond over-the-counter products you may use to fight acne (cleanser, exfoliant, disinfectant) you can also implement a few lifestyle changes that might help. Reducing stress, getting the appropriate amount of sleep, and exposing your skin to humidity can all work to minimize acne outbreaks.

Because acne is caused by excess oil that has been trapped in the dermis (which results in inflaming the area), exfoliating is a very important step in preventing and clearing up acne outbreaks. A particularly effective exfoliant for acne is salicylic acid because it penetrates the sebum, gets into the pores, and breaks up the oil. Because salicylic acid is an anti-inflammatory, it also acts to soothe the area and heal the inflammation more quickly. After cleansing and exfoliating you can disinfect the area with a topical treatment such as benzoyl peroxide.

PRODUCT RECOMMENDATIONS

CLEANSERS: non-foaming cleansers for daily use

- Dove Sensitive Skin Non-Foaming Cleanser
- Cetaphil Gentle Skin Cleanser
- Cetaphil Daily Facial Cleanser

EXFOLIANTS: exfoliants for weekly use

- Buf-Puf Extra Gentle Facial Sponge
- Buf-Puf Gentle Facial Sponge
- St. Ives Naturally Clear Apricot Scrub (for acne-prone skin)

MOISTURIZERS

- Aveeno Ultra-Calming Daily Moisturizer
- Neutrogena Healthy Skin Anti-Wrinkle Cream
- RevaléSkin Night Cream

SUNBLOCK

- EltaMD UV Facial SPF 30+
- Blue Lizard Australian Sunscreen–Face

Chapter 5

MAKEUP AND HAIRSTYLING

*"Kiss and make up—
but too much makeup has ruined many a kiss."*

—Mae West

As you walk through an art museum, you can't help but see the beauty of the art displayed on the wall. The subject tells a story and the palette of colors evokes a mood or an emotion. Wrapped around each of those pieces of art is a frame that enhances and defines the beauty. Sometimes the frame brings attention to a specific subject or color. The frame can also appear to change the relative size of a piece. A small frame for a large piece can enhance its size. Conversely, a large frame wrapped around a small piece will amplify its lack of breadth.

Your face is no different. The shape and flow of facial lines and prominences display your beauty and evoke emotion. The color and imperfections of your skin will also contribute or detract from your beauty in its entirety. And just like that piece of artwork with its frame, your face is framed and accentuated by your hair.

In this chapter, I will approach the art of facial beauty from another angle. In past chapters, I discussed ways to promote beauty by enhancing skin health while fighting the march of time. Future chapters will be dedicated to ways to surgically enhance and alter the shape and flow of those facial lines and prominences permanently. This chapter could aptly be called the art of camouflage. Hair care and makeup will not slow the aging process and will certainly not affect your face permanently. However, these temporary measures help define your best features while erasing, for a fleeting moment, those imperfections that otherwise detract from a beautiful piece of art.

THE ART OF MAKEUP

Makeup can be used to camouflage blemishes and deformities, enhance facial features, or project a mood (glamour, seduction, seriousness). Regardless of the purpose for applying makeup, good makeup application starts with correction of skin color. Most of our faces have some blotches and assorted pigmentation irregularities that can be minimized to improve facial appearance. A base, also called foundation, is effective for smoothing out skin color. The most important part of choosing a good base is deciding the level of opaqueness that is suitable for you. Base products can range from light to complete coverage.

Coverage Level	Product Types
light	tinted moisturizers
medium	creams, powders, water-based liquids
heavy	opaque bases, Dermablend-type products

You can achieve different results by combining different product levels. The most important tip is that thorough blending of bases is essential to give a seamless appearance. If in doubt, less is more to achieve a natural look with a healthy glow. Celebrity makeup artist Susan Ginsburg recommends, "If you are 35, use a light concealer with a water base, but at 75 neutralize the color by using a lighter color concealer in an oil base."

EYES AND EYEBROWS

Eyes are the windows to your soul. Eyes can reveal joy and sadness as well as distress. Eyes can flirt or seduce. No matter the situation, eyes and eyebrows are the most defining and distinguishing features of your face.

There are many opinions as to what shape of eye is ideal, but there are a few basic proportions that transcend cultural and generational differences. Beginning with the shape of the eye itself, an oval eye with the outer corner of the eye slightly higher than the inner corner is desirable. The lower eyelid should be horizontal with minimal bowing along the outer third of the eyelid. The lower lid should also be smooth, without bags, grooves, or shadows. The upper lid should be arched, with the peak of the arch at the border of the inner and middle thirds of the eye. The upper lid should be smooth, without excess folds of skin or bulges. The upper eyelid crease should be curved to parallel the curve of the border of the upper eyelid.

The eyebrow serves as a frame for the eye. The two components of the eyebrow are the brow and the oval of skin below the eyebrow (but not on the eyelid) above the outer third of the eye. The brow should be peaked along the border of the middle and outer third of the eye. If the peak is well placed, then the eyebrow skin oval will be well defined. The thickness of the brow is determined more by trends and cultural mores, but regardless of these trends, the shape of the eye and eyebrow remains constant.

The three main elements of eye makeup are eye shadow, mascara, and eyeliner.

Eye Shadow. There are many options when deciding how and why to use eye shadow. Traditional shadows are soft with neutral colors or light bronzes and are designed to enhance a natural look. For more evocative designs—to enhance a seductive look or to improve the shape of the eye—a dimensional appearance that involves multiple colors is ideal. If you opt for multicolored shadow, start with a cream base and then apply a second color in powder. When using any cream eye shadow, it is best to use as little as possible. For those for whom age has reduced the fold above the eye, you can create a virtual fold by shading in a crease on the upper eyelid with eyeliner. This can be best accomplished by starting the line from the outer corner of the upper eyelid and shading it in toward the middle.

Mascara. Eyelashes serve as a beacon that says, "Look at my eyes"—and mascara helps them send that message loud and clear. Mascara comes in forms that can lengthen, curl, thicken, or color your lashes. Choose wisely and apply carefully. The goal is to make your eyelashes look full but also

natural. Clumping of lashes together, or mascara that looks lumpy, is a defi-
nite no-no, and a sign that you used too much or did not wait between
applications for the previous application to dry. A recently FDA-approved
product called Latisse is capable of lengthening eyelashes by stimulating
natural eyelash growth without a need for daily mascara application.

Eyeliner. Eyeliner is the last tool to use in an effort to enhance the oval shape
of the eye. For many people with naturally beautiful eyes, eyeliner is overkill
and only serves to blur the lines between a beautiful look and a done or an
overdone look. However, for those without ideally oval-shaped eyes because
of age, genetics, or just plain luck, eyeliner can help create the appearance of
an almond-shaped eye. The best way to apply eyeliner is to pull the corner
of the eye outward to flatten out the eyelid margin and then apply the liner
from the inside to the outside corner of the eye. As with all makeup, use the
least possible product that will achieve the effect you are looking for. Too
much makeup will only serve to detract from, rather than enhance, your
natural beauty.

CHEEKS

The second most important feature on your face, in terms of beauty, may come as a
surprise. It is the cheek and surrounding area. Think of those beauties of the silver
screen, Charlize Theron or Grace Kelly. Both have exquisite cheeks that are full, adding
volume as well as width to their faces. The full cheek is something that has been defined
as desirable across cultures and trends. French barmaids in the seventeenth century
were the first to use blush, but tribal makeup has been employed to similar effect by
African women for more than a thousand years.

Makeup can enhance the cheek by creating contrast and shadow. The easiest way
to enhance the cheek is by applying a blush that matches the natural tone in your
cheeks when flush, while enhancing the contrast with a slightly darker shade of bronzer
below the cheek and on the jawline. You can also add a shimmer highlighter over the
blush to enhance the lifted appearance of your cheek. You can enhance the width of the

cheek and the entire face by applying darker bronzer to the sides of the nose, making it look narrower.

LIPS

After the eyes and cheeks, lips are the third most important feature on the face.

The ideal height ratio is 60 percent lower lip and 40 percent upper lip. The corners of the lips are slightly angled upward, and when a line is drawn through both corners, the line crosses the upper lip. As the lip ages, the upper lip becomes smaller, and vertical lines appear that cause bleeding of lipstick. You can use lip liner, lipstick, and lip gloss to create a balanced and sexy lip.

Big Lips. For the most part, big lips are desirable. They evoke a sexy, seductive appearance. However, as with anything, too much of a good thing is not too good! For big lips, always use muted colors—purples, browns, and bronzes—in your lipstick, so as not to overwhelm the natural beauty of the lips. Do not use too much gloss because that only gives the lips a larger appearance. For the fullest lips use a darker colored lipstick to make them appear smaller.

Small Lips. For small lips, several tricks can help make them look fuller. First, avoid dark colors, which tend to make lips appear smaller. To make them appear fuller, draw slightly beyond your lip border with a lip pencil or lip liner. Then apply lipstick, followed by white shadow on the center of the lips, over the lipstick. This look can be further enhanced with lip gloss.

Custom Lips. Sometimes the problem is not one of size but of shape. Angelina Jolie has a pouty fuller central upper lip, while Michelle Pfeiffer and Meg Ryan have made a career of having lips that are fuller on the outer thirds. Short of collagen or hyaluronic acid fillers (available in your dermatologist's office), you can use gloss to emphasize a shape. To make it pouty, emphasize the upper lip by applying gloss to the upper central lip. Conversely, apply the gloss on the outer thirds of the lip to look more like Meg.

Corrective Lip Camouflage. As we age, our lips lose volume and begin to wrinkle. Some of those wrinkles extend like rays of the sun from the red of the lip onto the skin surrounding the lips. As a result, lipstick can bleed into these wrinkles, emphasizing their presence and making you look older than desired. To stop lipstick from bleeding, use a lip liner over the lip first. The liner will hold the lipstick and stop the bleeding. For those with uneven lips, use a lighter colored lipstick on the smaller-sized lip to create the impression of volume.

Hair Color	Best Lipstick Colors
light blond	wine, berry, mauve
golden blond	coral, apricot, peach
blond/olive skin tones	peach, brown, terra-cotta
brunette	terra-cotta, cinnamon, darker red
red	peachy brown, cinnamon, terra-cotta

HAIR DESIGN AND YOUR FACE

Our hair frames our face, and the way it is cut should highlight your best features. Good haircuts include layering to enhance a feature like your cheeks, eyes, or lips. Layers should not fall too high (above your eyes) or above your ears. Length can be used to enhance a facial shape or compensate for a round or long face. The ideal length for hair should be at shoulder length, never longer. Longer lengths should be left for a teenage, younger look. If you desire a longer length for your hair, be careful to care for split ends and scraggly, frizzy ends. A classy way to have longer hair is to layer it in the back and allow it to come to a point between your shoulders.

Oval Face. An oval face is an ideal facial shape that can do well with most hairstyles. The key is to steer clear of any hairstyle that will detract from your ideal shape. Specifically, avoid too much volume on top of your head, which tends to make the face appear too long. A simple, surefire way to enhance an oval face is to create layers near the chin or cheekbone.

Round Face. In an effort to create an oval shape from a round or square face, adding height or length is desirable. Hampton's hairstylist Bianka Lefferts suggests that verticality can be enhanced by adding volume on top. Another way to add length is by creating bangs that start high on the forehead. The ideal cut for round or square faces would be a multilayered cut just below the chin. Avoid single-layer cuts.

Long Face. Just as with the round face, the desired goal for a long face is to make the face appear more oval. Obtaining a wider, more oval shape is achieved by adding width with long, side-sweeping bangs or a chin-length bob. Another great way to widen the face is by adding curls or waves to frame the face. Avoid hairstyles that add length.

PART TWO

Plastic Surgery Procedures

Chapter 6

LOWER FACE

"Some people, no matter how old they get, never lose their beauty—they merely move it from their faces into their hearts."

—Martin Buxbaum

B elieve it or not, 100 years have passed since the first facelift was performed and, no, Phyllis Diller was not the patient. But while the comedienne may not have been the first, her facelifts did represent a milestone in that they increased public awareness of using surgery to help people look younger. I should point out, since her transformation seemed to elicit more jeers than cheers, that surgical techniques have improved over the past 35 years. Now, rather than the problem of untested procedures, consumers have too many procedures from which to choose. Not only are there many types of facelifts, but the marketplace is currently flooded with a raft of "new and improved" procedures that may turn out to be neither. Adding to the confusion is the recent and troubling trend of practitioners who are not board-certified plastic surgeons performing procedures for which they have not been properly trained.

This chapter is designed to help you sift through all of your options, allowing you to make a clearheaded, educated decision about which procedures, if any, might be best for you. After all, any medical procedure is serious business and should be treated as such. My goal is to provide you with a detailed road map that will help you arrive at your desired destination—a rejuvenated you—with as few wasteful detours as possible.

ANATOMY AND AGING

To understand how a doctor can help you look younger, it is necessary to have a basic grasp of the anatomy of your face, and how getting older affects it. I will keep it simple, so there is no need to panic. But trust me when I say that educating yourself on the fundamentals of facial anatomy will greatly increase your comfort level when exploring the many medical options available to you.

There are four general anatomical components to your face and, contrary to popular belief, your skin is only part of the equation. It might help to think of your face as a building. The facade is what is visible from the outside, but it is by no means the only important element of that building. In fact, if the internal structure or foundation of the building becomes weak, then the facade will undoubtedly begin to show signs of trouble. The same is true of your face. That is why the lesser-known components of your facial anatomy are just as important as your skin when evaluating what needs to be done to rejuvenate your lower face.

SKIN

Healthy skin is an important element in looking your best. But no matter how well you take care of your skin, as you get older a number of processes will affect its appearance. Fundamental to these overall changes is that your cellular machinery is slowing down. Unfortunately, this means that your skin loses its ability to regenerate as quickly as it used to—if at all. For example, as the epidermis ages, it may no longer be able to exfoliate layers of dry, dead skin cells, which can result in a sallow appearance. (See chapters 2 and 4 for a review of the basic anatomy of your skin.)

In addition to the basic weakening of your cellular machinery, the two most notable changes to your aging skin are the loss of elastin and collagen. With less elastin it is more difficult for stretched skin to return to its original shape or for wrinkles to smooth themselves out. And a loss of collagen leads to thinning skin that is more prone to fine lines and wrinkles as well as an overall crepey look.

There are three types of wrinkles that can occur during the aging process. Plastic surgeons make a distinction among the three because, even if they may look the same, their root causes are different. And this means they are often corrected using different procedures.

Gravitational Wrinkles. As you age, gravity pulls down the skin of your face. Genetics and skin type may determine the degree to which you will be affected by gravity, but there is no doubt your skin will start to sag. Certain areas are especially prone to gravity, including the marionette lines around your mouth and the skin on your neck. It should be noted that gravitational wrinkles are the easiest wrinkles to surgically correct.

Dynamic Wrinkles. These wrinkles are caused by the muscles in your face. Every time you frown, smile, or raise an eyebrow your facial muscles are moving your skin from its resting position. These repetitive movements— day after day and year after year—cause damage to the skin lying above these overworked facial muscles, most notably on your forehead and around your mouth. Dynamic wrinkles become even more likely as you age because of a loss of elastin and collagen, making it harder for this damage to be repaired.

Conformational Wrinkles. As the name implies, these wrinkles are caused by your skin conforming to a certain shape after repeated movement. However, unlike dynamic wrinkles, conformational wrinkles are not caused by the actual muscle under the skin, but rather just by the movement. Your neck area, where it bends up and down, is most prone to conformational wrinkling. As we age, these wrinkles can become more pronounced because of more years of this repetition and because of the loss of elastin and collagen. It is important to note that these types of folds are difficult to get rid of; even if attempts are made to fill them in or smooth them out under the skin, any outward improvement is minimal.

SOFT TISSUE OR ADIPOSE LAYER

Directly under your skin is a layer of fat that provides important contours to your face. The good news is that, unlike most areas of your body where fat is not particularly welcome, the right amount of facial fat actually makes you more beautiful. It softens the angles of your face and helps your features flow more smoothly into one another. Fat also creates that full, nicely rounded cheek or voluptuously shaped lip that so many people covet. Over time the amount of soft tissue you have in your face may change, affecting the way you look as you age.

A loss of facial fat can result in harsh, angular features or a hollowed-out look, both of which can amplify the effects of aging. Adding to the problem is that as facial volume decreases, the remaining structural components may start to sag (think of a deflating balloon). Conversely, while weight gain can hide finer facial wrinkles, it may cause deeper wrinkles and folds at the neck or jowls as your skin tries to accommodate the increased volume. Both increased and decreased facial volume can be dealt with surgically: A hollow face can be filled with implants, fat injections, or one of the many types of filler on the market, while excess jowls can be lifted or reduced in size through surgery.

I should point out that overall excess weight in the facial area—from any cause— has the potential to diminish the results of a facelift. No matter what procedure a surgeon performs, too much facial volume in certain areas is going to create grooves, folds, and deep wrinkles that will take away from any positive results. Just one more reason to watch your weight!

SMAS

If we return to our building analogy, the most important structural element of your face is the submusculoaponeurotic system, usually referred to as the SMAS. Located between the bones of your face and the fat under your skin, the SMAS is made up of muscle and connective tissue (including fascia and fascial bands) that comprise the structural foundation of your face. While the SMAS is a distinct layer that is somewhat free-floating, it is attached to your skin and bone in a few critical places (at the cheek, for example). Two important components of your SMAS are:

Fascia. The best way to describe fascia is to think of a steak. If you look closely at a sirloin you will see tentacle-like white gristle that seems to hold the meat together. Fascia is similar to that steak gristle. It is the connective tissue that envelopes, separates, and binds the different soft structures of your face into a whole. Like all other elements I have discussed, aging affects the fascia as well. Most important, the loss of elastin makes it more difficult for fascia to bind soft tissue like it did when you were younger. This can lead to an overall saggy, elongated appearance.

Muscle. There are 27 distinct muscles in your face. While I am not going to discuss each one individually, it is important to say a few general words about them. As mentioned above, the SMAS contains muscles (and fascia) that act to perform a variety of functions—most notably holding your face together and providing you with the ability to communicate through facial animation. When you age, muscles that have been stretched over and over again lose their ability to bounce back—yet another problem due to the loss of elastin. And as facial muscles lose their strength, your entire SMAS will start to sag.

Since your SMAS does most of the "heavy lifting" in keeping your face young-looking, when it starts to go the outward signs tend to be quite noticeable. Other aging processes that affect the skin, such as exposure to the sun or loss of collagen, usually result in fine lines and wrinkles. But when the SMAS weakens you will start to see deeper grooves and furrows around your mouth and eyes. This is because as the SMAS sags, so does the skin and fat that it has been supporting over the years.

Unlike the many preventative measures that can be taken to slow the effects of aging on your skin, there are no topical treatments that can protect your SMAS from the ravages of time. As with all aging tissue, free radicals build up in your SMAS and weaken the cellular processes that keep the muscles and fascia taut. Antioxidants will certainly slow the aging process but cannot stop it. That's the bad news. The good news is that a gifted plastic surgeon can work on your SMAS to create a natural-looking face-lift (a result that cannot be achieved by simply manipulating the skin). So, while your SMAS might cause more noticeable signs of aging, it also provides an opportunity for great surgical results. More on this later.

BONE

The saying "use it or lose it" is particularly applicable to your teeth and jaw. As you age, the stress needed to keep your teeth healthy will tend to diminish, and you can start to lose bone mass. As your facial bones lose mass your jaw rotates upward, which has the unfortunate effect of making your teeth appear shorter. Believe it or not, studies show that our ideal of youthful beauty is based on, among other things, 2 millimeters of teeth being visible when your mouth is slightly open and relaxed. When your jaw rotates upward it conceals more of your teeth behind your lips, making your teeth appear shorter. And while this change is more subtle than sagging skin or fat, it tends to amplify the overall look of aging. (More on this in chapter 7.)

The table on the next page outlines what can be done to correct changes to your face due to aging.

I'M STARTING TO LOOK OLD!

Now that I have gone over the basics of your facial anatomy and how aging affects each component, it should be easier to understand the varied surgical options being offered today and which procedures may be right for you. When considering a facelift you will be asked to make two distinct decisions: the areas of your face you would like treated and the type of surgery the doctor will employ. While the old adage "a million ways to skin a cat" may sound a bit too close for comfort here, the point could not be truer when discussing plastic surgery and, more specifically, facelifts.

As in any professional field, opinions differ among plastic surgeons as to how to achieve the best results. So while the goal may be the same—making you look younger—the techniques used by plastic surgeons can be quite different. There are pros and cons to each, and you should weigh them carefully when considering a facelift. As I have emphasized before, any procedure you choose is major surgery and should not be taken lightly.

While there are many criteria that should be examined when choosing the right doctor (a topic covered at length in chapter 12), this is a good time to emphasize one in particular when discussing differing surgical techniques. *Always* ask to look at "after" photographs taken at least a year following the surgery. This is important because some procedures can produce results that are initially unstable. For example,

	Skin	Fat	SMAS	Bone
Components	dermis, epidermis	fat, fascial bands	muscle, fascia, nerve fibers	jawbone, teeth
Signs of Aging	fine wrinkles, coarse wrinkles, rough skin, blotchy pigmented skin, thinning crepey skin	sagging of fat, loss of fat volume, gain of fat volume in undesirable areas	jowls, marionette lines, turkey gobbler neck, nasolabial folds	loss of bone volume, loss of teeth, shortening of the face
Causes of Aging	sun, pollution, smoking, poor diet, genetics (cellular aging), gravity, repetitive muscle movement	cellular aging, gravity, repetitive muscle movement, large weight shifts	cellular aging, gravity, repetitive muscle movement	loss of bone volume as a result of trauma or tooth loss
Treatment Options	antioxidants, retinoids, skin bleaches, fruit acids, surgery, chemical peels, lasers	surgical lifting of fat, surgical adding or removing of fat, fillers	surgical tightening procedures for the SMAS (facelift)	dental correction of oral deficiencies, cheek and chin implants, bone grafts

the subperiosteal facelift can cause severe swelling that may not subside for close to a year, obscuring the true results of the facelift during that time. And a skin-only facelift can stretch skin so it looks good immediately following the procedure, only to sag back to its presurgery position a year later (a rather common result in older patients due to diminished elasticity). In both cases, a photo taken two months after the procedure is not going to give you an accurate indication of the success or failure of that surgery. So don't be shy—make sure your doctor is showing you "after" photos taken at least a year following the surgery!

A surgeon's "after" photographs should show a noticeable yet *natural* improvement in overall appearance. When studying the photo book you do not want to see an older patient who suddenly looks 20 years younger. The goal of any gifted surgeon is to subtly rejuvenate a patient without making drastic changes. In addition to notable

I can't tell you how often, during an initial consultation, a patient will ask me, "What do you think I need, Dr. Freund?" Plastic surgery is usually elective and beauty is subjective—a combination that makes it both irresponsible and dangerous for me to answer that question. One of the first things I explain to my patients is that, as a plastic surgeon, it is my job to help you discover what you want. I cannot possibly understand what it means to be you, how you feel about yourself, what you like—and don't like—about your appearance. Nor would I dare to guess. What any good doctor should do is lead you through a series of questions to help clarify what your goals and expectations are regarding plastic surgery. Only then will you and your doctor be able to achieve the most natural-looking results that fit properly into the context of your life—and your face! By the way, if your doctor does answer that question, I would look for another doctor.

caveat emptor

improvements, you should also be mindful of what I call the "Five Telltale Signs of a Bad Facelift," listed below. While some are quite visible in photographs, others may be more easily concealed. So make a point of looking at close-ups of the ears (behind and in front) as well as the hairline.

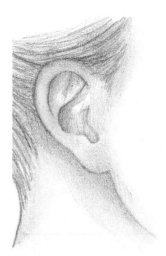

"NORMAL" EAR/SIDEBURN

Pixie Ears. The best facelifts do not place excessive tension on the incision line, especially around the ear and earlobe. If too much tension is placed on the bottom of the earlobe, the lobe will be pulled downward and across the face in an unnatural manner, called a pixie ear.

Nike Swoop. We all know the trademark swoop on the side of a Nike sneaker. That same swoop can appear on your face if a surgeon pulls the soft tissue of your face out toward the ears. While your cheekbone supports the upper cheek and your jawbone supports the jawline, the area between the two (where your teeth are) is slightly recessed. When soft tissue is pulled out toward the ear that recessed space becomes more of a pronounced indentation, what I call a "swoop."

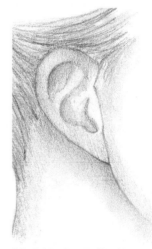

SIGNS OF A BAD FACELIFT: PIXIE EARS

The earlobe is pulled down and forward on the face as a result of too much tension put on the skin in that area.

Loss of Sideburn. Good surgeons recognize the importance of maintaining the hairline and have techniques to keep your natural sideburn in its proper position. If a less-than-capable surgeon pulls your skin up and away from the middle part of your face your sideburns can rise as well. Needless to say, this becomes a serious

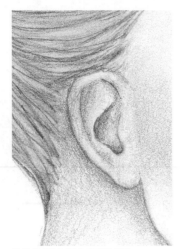

SIGNS OF A BAD FACELIFT:
LOSS OF SIDEBURN

Older facelift techniques pull up the sideburn, and for some patients that may result in a loss of the sideburn and hair at the temple as well.

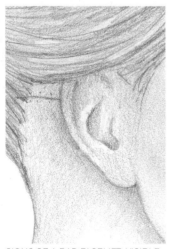

SIGNS OF A BAD FACELIFT: VISIBLE SCARRING BEHIND THE EAR

Older techniques also would pull the hair behind the ears, leaving a wide swath of skin behind the ear where hair normally resides. Another component of poor technique behind the ear leaves a visible scar.

problem for active women who need to pull their hair back.

Postauricular Scarring (Scars Behind the Ear). For the majority of facelift patients, the scar behind the ear is usually extended into the hair in order the get the best results in the neck area. Many surgeons leave scars that are quite obvious, making it difficult for a postoperative patient to pull her hair back in a ponytail. Good surgeons have ways to hide these scars. Sometimes these procedures will also pull the hairline behind the ear too far backward, leaving an unnatural bald spot behind the ear.

Ugly Scars at Front of Ear. Some surgeons still leave a scar near the front of the ear even though new techniques allow for scars to be completely concealed inside the ear canal. One warning—if this technique is not done correctly, the tragus (the bump of cartilage at the front of the ear canal) can be distorted. In addition, this new technique is not appropriate for men because they need to shave the pulled skin that now extends onto the tragus.

Even before making an initial consultation with a plastic surgeon you will need to evaluate your goals and expectations. Do you think the loose skin on your neck is the problem? Or perhaps you would like to correct those folds between your nose and mouth? Whatever the case may be, in order to identify the area of your face that may need attention you will find a helpful illustrated guide at the end of this chapter. Once you have evaluated your face you can then discuss the trouble spots with your doctor and go over which procedures are likely to give you the most bang for the buck. I am not simply referring to dollars here, since most people lead busy lives and their recuperation time is also a consideration.

I very often employ a Chinese-menu approach when assessing how best to rejuvenate a patient's face. This involves designing a customized program using a variety of procedures and very often working on different areas of the face during one session. The term may sound funny in a book on plastic surgery, but there is an important underlying concept to it. In selecting only the menu items that you feel are needed, your facelift will be right for *you*. My Chinese-menu approach offers another important benefit, however unintended. A doctor should never lose sight of the whole, and by working on different areas of the face at the same time the delicate interdependency of each component becomes a constant consideration—which can only improve your results.

To understand what a facelift can and cannot do, let's take an imaginary trip to your local tailor. Say you have a pair of baggy, wrinkled trousers that are too big for you. The tailor would use chalk, pins, thread, and a needle to resize the trousers so they fit you again. Further, if the trousers had a lining, that would be taken in as well. A plastic surgeon working on your face is essentially doing the same thing the tailor is doing to your pants. In particular, a good plastic surgeon is mindful of the various layers of your face just as a good tailor is mindful of the lining in the pants. But what about those annoying wrinkles—do they simply disappear because the trousers have been altered? No, the tailor would remove the big wrinkles by taking in the pants to fit you properly and press the fabric to remove the fine wrinkles. Your skin is no different. After a facelift a plastic surgeon very often suggests a trip to a cosmetic dermatologist, who is better equipped to handle those fine lines and wrinkles (see chapter 3).

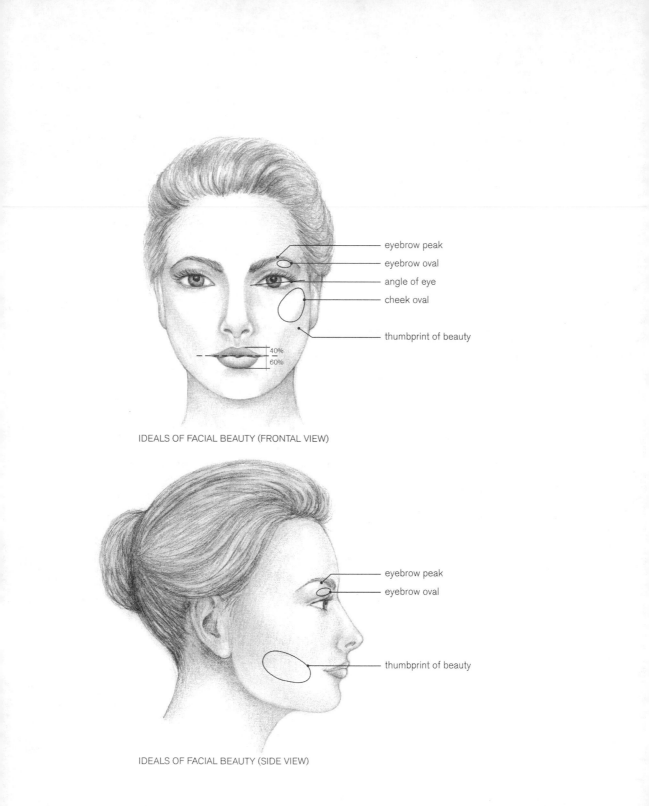

IDEALS OF FACIAL BEAUTY (FRONTAL VIEW)

eyebrow peak
eyebrow oval
angle of eye
cheek oval
thumbprint of beauty
40%
60%

IDEALS OF FACIAL BEAUTY (SIDE VIEW)

eyebrow peak
eyebrow oval
thumbprint of beauty

IDEALS OF FACIAL BEAUTY

Working within the parameters discussed in chapter 1, there are certain universals that I use when assessing a patient's options for maximizing the benefits of any rejuvenating surgery.

Eyebrows are one of the most important features of an attractive face. The ideal eyebrow starts over the inner corner of the eye and angles up to reach a peak on the outside one-third of the eyeball. Then the eyebrow softly angles downward for its remaining length. This ideally arched eyebrow allows for an oval area of skin below the peak but above the eyelid.

The eyes should be oval-shaped and angled slightly upward toward the outer corner of the eye. The upper eyelid should be arched, with the peak toward the inner eye, while the lower eyelid should be bowed with the lowest point toward the outer corner of the eye.

The cheeks are perhaps as important as the eyes and brows. They should be large ovals that extend from below the eyes upward and outward to occupy the area outside the eye. A full cheek will create a three-dimensional contour with smooth flowing lines, diminishing any sharp angles of the face.

Below the cheek there should be a slightly hollowed-out area that flows to a fuller jawline, which should be oval-shaped. This hollow area between the cheek and jaw is called the "thumbprint of beauty."

Lips should be full and shapely, with the lower lip being slightly larger than the upper lip in a 60:40 ratio. The corners of the lips should be upturned so that an imaginary line drawn between the two would pass through the upper lip. The lower lip can have an oval fullness across the entire lip. The upper lip has fullness on either side of the midline, resembling two separate ovals.

Finally, the proportion of **the nose** should fit on the face in size and angle and should have flowing lines. Although many people worry about their noses incessantly, ironically the nose is perhaps the least important feature when identifying a beautiful person.

WHAT ARE MY CHOICES?

Now that you understand the basic anatomy of your face and have a sense of the general ideals of beauty outlined above, you are better equipped to choose the procedure most appropriate for your own rejuvenation. So let's get started.

THE "LIFESTYLE FACELIFT" (SKIN-ONLY FACELIFT)

It is fitting to begin our discussion with the skin-only facelift because it was the first type of facelift ever performed—more than 100 years ago. As the name implies, this procedure involves manipulating only the skin in order to make you look younger. The most obvious benefit of this type of facelift is that it is the simplest procedure available. And with simplicity comes fewer possible surgical complications, a shortened recovery time, and results that may be visible more quickly.

Incisions are made near each ear (the exact location would depend upon, among other things, the amount of excess skin being removed, the patient's hairline, and the contours of the patient's face) and the skin is pulled away from the center of the face and reattached at the incision. In the hands of a good surgeon—and with the right patient—the outcome can be positive. However, because the skin is reattached in a "stretched" position, a certain amount of elasticity is required or the results will not last very long. Since skin progressively loses elasticity with age, this procedure should not be considered by anyone over the age of 50 because the stretched skin will start to sag—not the desired result after a facelift!

Another potential problem with this procedure goes back to our trousers analogy. Remember the SMAS—that important layer of muscle and connective tissue located between your skin and bone? The SMAS is like the lining of the trousers. A skin-only facelift is the equivalent of a tailor taking in the pants while ignoring the lining. Most would agree that those altered pants would look considerably better if the lining were taken in as well. The same is true of your skin, possibly even more so since the SMAS is an important part of the machinery that controls facial animation and expression. When their doctor ignores their sagging SMAS and fatty layer above it, some skin-only facelift patients can end up looking a bit wooden and taut.

Which brings us to another possible problem with a skin-only facelift: the "Nike Swoop" I mentioned in my list of five telltale signs of a bad facelift. This mistake has been immortalized by a certain well-known celebrity who could be the star of "Plastic Surgery Gone Bad." When looking at her face it is clear that her skin has been stretched too tightly in a horizontal direction, accentuating that hollow between her jaw and cheekbone. Since this would never occur naturally, it is obvious she has had a facelift— and a bad one at that. If you are considering a lifestyle lift it is important to discuss with your doctor the direction in which your skin is going to be pulled. The best results come from a vertical pull.

Finally, with all of the advances made in medical knowledge, technique, and equipment over the past 100 years, it seems a bit backward to opt for a procedure that has hardly changed in as much time, even if it is currently being repackaged as something "new and improved." That is not to say positive results cannot be achieved with a skin-only facelift under the right circumstances, especially when a gifted surgeon is doing it. But I feel it is important to point out the limitations of the procedure.

SMAS FACELIFT

Introduced in 1974 by Dr. Tord Skoog of Sweden, the SMAS facelift represented a major leap forward in achieving more natural-looking results. The breakthrough concept of the SMAS facelift was to manipulate the skin and SMAS separately, a technique that has been improved over the past 30 years. Since both your skin and your SMAS sag during the aging process, it logically follows that lifting both will provide you with a more complete facelift. In fact, lifting the SMAS is usually considered more important than lifting the skin because it is the sagging SMAS that weighs down your skin in the first

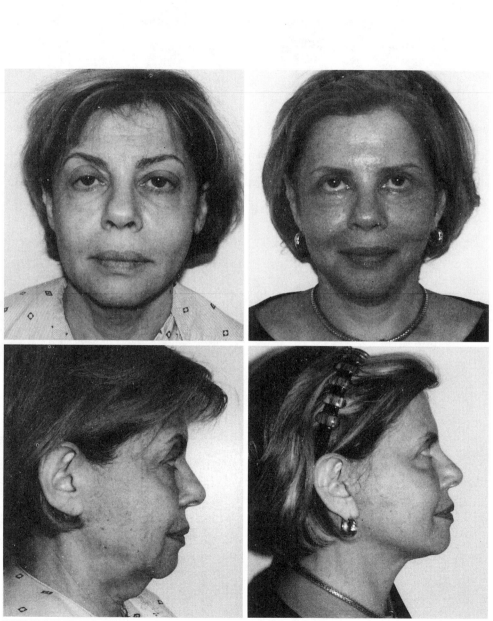

50-YEAR-OLD FEMALE WITH A SMAS FACELIFT

place. Very often the extra, saggy skin that was so noticeable prior to surgery simply disappears on its own after a good SMAS facelift. A well-executed SMAS facelift offers results that plastic surgeons have been after for 100 years—lifting your face without changing its contour or shape.

Remember those trousers that needed taking in and how the lining, too, had to be altered in order for them fit properly again? The SMAS facelift is the surgical equivalent of altering the lining. The surgeon separates the skin from the SMAS, lifts the two layers individually, and then pulls each—often in slightly different directions—to give you a smoother, younger look. And because the SMAS is hidden under your skin, it can be stitched in locations on your face other than the skin incision near your ear. This has a number of benefits. It allows your surgeon more leeway in finding the optimum places to anchor the pulled tissue, the SMAS can be pulled toward your cheek (vertically) rather than your ear (laterally) helping to avoid the infamous "Nike Swoop," and it diminishes the potential of an overly taut result because the SMAS is being repositioned upward, not outward.

Beyond the most important benefit of achieving natural-looking results, the SMAS facelift offers some other positives that are worth mentioning. For example, because the skin is not stretched excessively, the results tend to last longer and won't droop in a year (remember, aging skin has less elasticity and does not respond well to being stretched). Additionally, the SMAS facelift is a good choice for all ages—younger women whose skin is not showing many signs of aging yet and older women whose skin is less elastic. Finally, it is my opinion that the SMAS facelift offers patients the best ratio between optimal results and minimal risk of doing any damage—a consideration that should be taken seriously when discussing any surgery.

There are a few risks associated with a SMAS facelift. The large amount of dissection (separating the two layers from each other) can result in the formation of a hematoma—a collection of blood below the skin. Although this tends to be more of

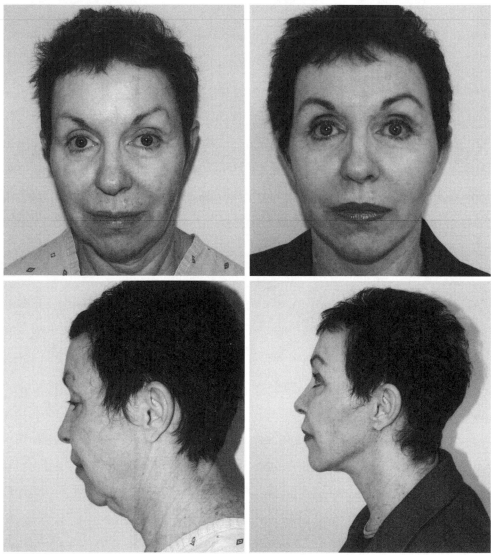

52-YEAR-OLD FEMALE WITH SMAS FACELIFT

a nuisance rather than a serious health threat, the standard postoperative regimen of reduced facial movement, limited exertion, and meticulous blood pressure control can help prevent this problem from developing. There can also be some nerve damage as a result of manipulating the SMAS. However, this is very rare and, if it were to happen, the nerve injury is usually temporary.

DEEP PLANE FACELIFT

While both your skin and your SMAS are manipulated during a deep plane facelift (as in a SMAS facelift), there is one critical difference between the two procedures. During a deep plane facelift, the surgeon does *not* separate the skin from the SMAS. Rather, the two layers are pulled together in the same direction, toward incisions near your ear or hairline. Doctors who perform these facelifts believe the results are more durable because the blood supply from the underlying SMAS is still attached to the skin. However, there is no evidence that suggests this is true.

Although the goal of this chapter is to present the various facelift options in a balanced manner, I find it difficult to remain neutral about the deep plane facelift. My primary concern with this procedure is that it is extremely invasive. Remember the last point I made about the SMAS facelift—that it offers patients the best ratio between optimal results and minimal risks? My opinion is that the deep plane facelift puts the patient at greater risk for nerve damage and excessive swelling without offering any benefits unique to this procedure. The mantra for cosmetic surgery, which is elective, should always be *"primum no nocerum,"* or, in plain English, "First and foremost, do no harm."

Unlike the skin-only and SMAS facelifts, a surgeon needs to put an enormous amount of stress on the connective tissue of the face in order to pull both layers—together—toward the ear. If you think of an unmade bed with different layers to it, the challenges of a deep plane facelift become apparent. No one would try to smooth out the crumpled top bedspread by simply pulling on the sheets below. In fact, if the sheets were being pulled harder and harder in an attempt to straighten out the bedspread they might actually come loose from the mattress. I am not suggesting that a surgeon could pull so hard during a deep plane facelift that your skin and SMAS would be torn from your face. Rather, I am trying to illustrate how a "second generation" pull requires more stress while delivering diminished results.

Another potential problem with the deep plane facelift is that it demands more dissection. For a surgeon to loosen that layer of skin and SMAS in a way that allows it to be pulled and manipulated as a single sheet, the cuts have to be considerably more invasive than with any other type of facelift. In a deep plane facelift the only way to pull or lift any part of the SMAS is to dissect it, along with the skin, all the way from your ear down to your nose or mouth. Compare this to the dissections of a SMAS facelift, which are only a few centimeters long because the surgeon has lifted the skin off the SMAS, and you will begin to understand the difference in trauma between the two. In a deep plane facelift the considerable dissection not only causes severe swelling for up to a year, but the swelling can be a potential problem *during* the surgery. If there is an hour or two lag between the time the doctor works on the two sides of your face (which is a very real possibility) then the swelling of the first side can get in the way of a doctor's ability to gauge the correct balance and symmetry of your face while completing the surgery.

The last, but certainly not the least, of my concerns regarding the deep plane facelift is the potential for nerve damage. Because of the large dissections as well as the stress needed to pull the SMAS and skin together, there is a very real chance that some of the many nerves in your face will be permanently damaged. Of course no surgeon goes into a procedure thinking this will happen, but the truth is that it does happen and at a higher rate than with any of the other procedures discussed. Do you want to be the patient this happens to? Even on the smallest scale, nerve damage to the face would change the way you look—forever.

In conclusion, I think that the risks of the deep plane facelift outweigh the benefits. What's more, these risks are unnecessary since there are other procedures able to give you the same—if not better—results.

SUBPERIOSTEAL FACELIFT

Right above the bones of the face is a fascia-like layer called the periosteum. As the name suggests, a surgeon performing a subperiosteal facelift gets very close to the bone and lifts all of the layers (the skin, fatty tissue, SMAS, and periosteum) together. There are benefits to the subperiosteal facelift, primary among them that it is performed with an endoscope (a tiny camera attached to a small tube), which allows for smaller incisions and a generally less-invasive procedure. Think of the endoscope as a scout. It surveys the territory and sends back images—via the camera—so the surgeon can make small incisions at the most optimal places and do the lifting and pulling at those localized areas on your face. Another benefit of the subperiosteal facelift, in contrast to the deep plane facelift, is that the pulling of the different layers is being done well below the nerves, thereby minimizing the risk of nerve damage. Finally, the blood supply is not overly disturbed with this facelift, which usually results in less swelling and swelling that goes away more quickly.

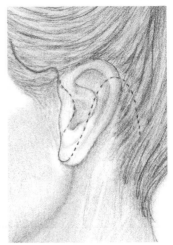

FULL FACELIFT INCISION

The typical incision runs from the sideburn, in front of the ear, then wraps behind the ear and finishes in the hair behind the ear. Newer techniques hide the scar inside the ear canal, instead of in front of the ear. (Both incisions are demonstrated in this picture.)

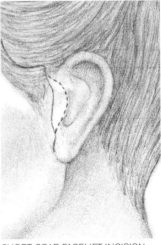

SHORT-SCAR FACELIFT INCISION

The incision used for midface lifts and limited facelifts eliminates the incision behind the ear, leaving only a scar in the sideburn and in front of the ear.

The primary downside of subperiosteal facelift—and it is not a minor one—is that because the pulling and lifting are done deep in the tissue of your face, the results often turn out to be less noticeable. Remember the unmade bed analogy I used regarding the deep plane facelift where I described it as a "second generation" pull? Well, the subperiosteal facelift is a "third generation" pull, the equivalent of pulling the mattress pad in the hopes that the bedspread—the top layer—will miraculously smooth itself out. The subperiosteal facelift works on the premise of indirect stress. It is a procedure purposely designed to work farther from the top layers of your face (the skin and SMAS) in order to achieve what are touted as its primary three benefits—quicker recovery times, smaller scars, and less trauma to the face. But I am sorry to report that because of those very aims a somewhat diminished end result is part of the equation. At its best, the subperiosteal facelift is most useful for cheek lifts for younger patients.

	Skin-only Lift	SMAS Lift	Deep Plane Lift	Subperiosteal Lift
Incision Site	short scar	short scar or full facelift scar	short scar or full facelift scar	temple or sideburn scar
Plane of Dissection	under the skin	under skin and partly under SMAS	under SMAS only	under periosteum
Durability	short	long	long	long
Swelling	minimal	moderate	severe, up to one year	moderate
Correction of Cheek Sagging	mild	excellent	moderate	moderate
Correction of Marionette Lines and Jowls	mild	excellent	good	poor
Tightening of the Skin	good	best	moderate	poor
Hematoma	rare	2–4%	1–3%	rare
Nerve Injury	rare	<1%	1–3%	rare
Overall Natural Result	moderate	excellent if done well with vertical lift of SMAS	good	good

THREAD LIFTS

I almost opted to exclude any discussion of thread lifts because I do not think they are going to be available much longer. But since some surgeons are still performing them I thought it important to explain how thread lifts work and why they are not a reliable option for lower face rejuvenation.

The concept behind thread lifts is simple enough. Threads with tiny barbs (think of really small fish hooks) are run through the soft tissue under your skin, pulling it up as it goes. When the correct amount of lift has been achieved, the three to four threads are anchored near your temple with the idea that they will hold your SMAS and skin in place and create a younger look. The main selling point for thread lifts has been that they are less invasive and thus carry fewer risks than traditional facelift options.

That may be true, but thread lifts don't work. The threads are just not strong enough to hold things in place over time. Regular facial movements as well as gravity weaken them and everything starts to sag back to its original position. Even worse is when only one or two of the threads weaken, creating a particularly lopsided, freakish look. So in my opinion thread lifts should go the way of the eight-track tape and be taken off the market.

CHOOSING A FACELIFT PROCEDURE

As has been made apparent, there are pros and cons to each of the above facelift procedures. Deciding which type of facelift is best for you will depend on your specific needs, your age, your expectations, and what your doctor recommends. The good news is that after reading this chapter you are now prepared to ask the right questions when meeting with your plastic surgeon. This allows you to weigh your options in an educated and deliberate manner so that you end up with the procedure that gives you the best results.

If you were wondering which type of facelift I most often perform, it is the SMAS facelift. I find it offers my patients the most balanced ratio between minimal risk and optimal results. If for some strange reason I could not perform a SMAS facelift my

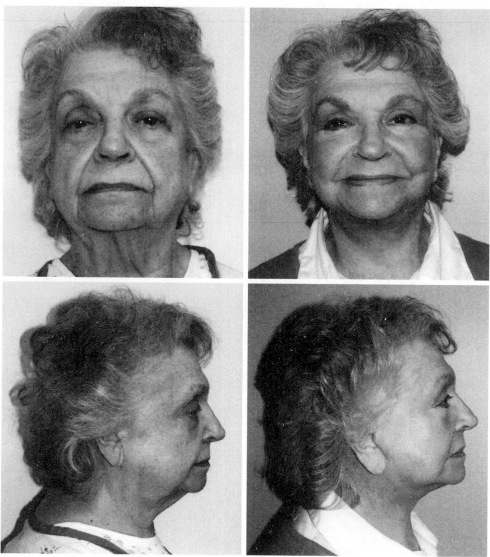

82-YEAR-OLD FEMALE WITH SMAS FACELIFT

second choice would be the subperiosteal facelift since it, too, represents a (slightly less) balanced ratio between minimized risk and optimized results. The skin-only facelift, in my opinion, is outdated; while it carries minimal risk, it does not provide particularly impressive results. I would not perform a deep plane facelift under any circumstances as I think the risk of nerve damage, although still quite minimal, is just too great.

A few things to be aware of when interviewing doctors while considering a facelift:

Take note of the amount of time allotted for your surgery. Too little time (1 to 2 hours) could mean that your surgeon is not going to be present for the entire procedure, or, worse yet, rush through your facelift. Too much time (6 to 7 hours) may be a signal that your doctor is still learning. Not only is that not who you want to do your surgery, but being under the knife for that long can lead to excessive swelling, which, in itself, is just not a good thing. The optimal time allotted should be about 2 to 4 hours.

Avoid gimmicky advertising. If a doctor is using words like "cosmetic surgeon" or "facial plastic surgery" it is usually a tipoff that this doctor is not a board-certified plastic surgeon. Your face is too important to trust to someone who has not had plastic surgical training. And no matter what that practitioner may say, there is a reason plastic surgeons are board certified.

Don't be oversold. There is nothing more suspect than a plastic surgeon who suggests he can "fix" things that you have not asked about. One of the aspects of my practice that I am most proud of is my ability to say no to patients, which any good doctor must be able to do. I consider it even more egregious if a doctor actually tries to sell you on a procedure you weren't interested in from the start. My advice to you is to run out of that office as fast as you can!

"Before" and "after" photos. As I have already mentioned, it is important that you are looking at "before" and "after" photos of patients that will actually tell you something about the doctor's skills. So make certain that the "after" photos you are looking at were taken at least a year following the surgery. This allows the results to settle and provide you with an accurate assessment of the results.

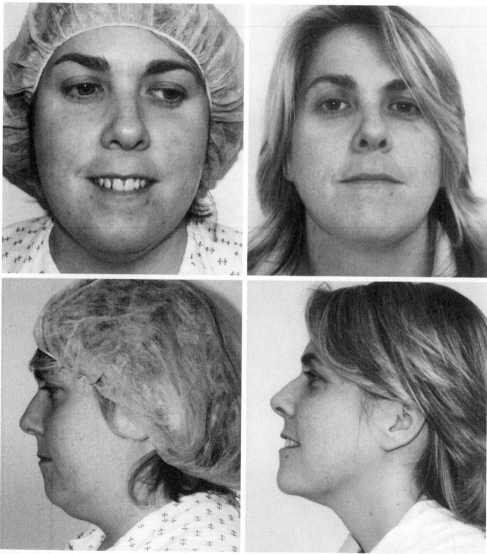

36-YEAR-OLD FEMALE WITH NECK LIPOSUCTION

THE NECK

If you are uncomfortable with the way your neck looks you have probably found creative ways to conceal it, but your wardrobe of scarves and turtlenecks has its limits—especially during the summer months! When the first signs of aging start to present themselves, many of my patients become particularly concerned with the neck area. The good news is that your neck can be beautifully rejuvenated through a variety of surgical procedures. These can be performed either alone or in conjunction with a facelift, depending on what you and your doctor decide.

The three anatomical factors affecting how your neck looks as you age are fat deposits, aging platysma bands, and excess or sagging skin.

PROBLEM: FAT; SOLUTION: LIPOSUCTION

Regardless of a patient's weight, I have found that most people gain some fat in their neck as they get older. The most effective procedure for getting rid of this fat is liposuction. Of course, if a lot of fat is removed and you have poor skin elasticity, liposuction has solved one problem but created another—excess skin. Thus, very often neck liposuction is performed in concert with either skin redraping or a more involved procedure that actually cuts out the extra skin. How can you gauge if you are a candidate for

caveat emptor

> The neck area is the only place on the face that liposuction should be performed. Some physicians try to sculpt the face by liposuction, but this poses several problems. First, facial muscles that are responsible for conveying emotion and facial animation can be disrupted by liposuction, leading to strange or distorted facial movements. Second, many people lose volume in their faces due to aging. Thus, removing additional volume through liposuction anywhere on the face except the neck will only amplify an aged look.

liposuction alone? A simple rule of thumb is that if you are a nonsmoker and younger than 40 you are likely a good candidate for liposuction alone. If you are over 50 you will probably require additional procedures to address the issue of sagging skin. For those who fall into the in-between category (ages 40 to 50), the best way to be sure of what you need is to consult with a plastic surgeon.

> While loss of fat more often presents itself around the cheekbone, some people can lose fat in their neck area as they age, leading to a skeletal look. The only option to correct this problem is the use of fat injections. A surgeon harvests fat from your body and then injects it into the area that needs filling. Since fat is live tissue it must be harvested and injected during the same session. Beware of anyone telling you it can be frozen and reinjected over different sessions, because it won't work. Someday that might be the case, but the technology just is not there yet.
>
> *caveat emptor*

PROBLEM: PLATYSMA BANDS; SOLUTIONS: BOTOX AND PLATYSMAPLASTY

Platysma bands (which are a muscle) extend from the outer edge of your jawbone all the way down your neck, holding most of its soft tissue in place. Using an analogy to better understand how these bands work, let's say you are taking a nap in a hammock and your friends decide to pull a prank by wrapping both ends more tightly around each tree. What would it feel like when you awoke? No doubt, the hammock would be much more taut and your body would now feel constricted within it. Taking things to an uncomfortable—and unrealistic—extreme, if the hammock were to be tightened like a vise, your body would probably just pop out of it and land on the ground below. This is basically what happens to the soft tissue of your lower face when your platysma bands start to move and widen with age. Further complicating this situation is that these bands have a natural split at the horizontal center of your neck to accommodate the thyroid gland. And it is at this opening that soft tissue starts to escape from widening platysma bands, creating what most of us refer to as a "turkey gobbler neck" or "wattles." Thankfully, there are number of procedures that are effective in correcting this problem.

Botox can be injected to paralyze the platysma bands so they relax and become less taut. This works well on younger patients who have only moderate platysmal band problems. The benefit of a nonsurgical solution is obvious, but keep in mind that Botox is only effective when there is a minimal amount of widening and the condition of the skin is still good. Of course, another issue with Botox is that it wears off and needs to be reinjected every three to six months. Still, it is worth mentioning because with the right patient it can be a cost-effective, noninvasive solution to beginning problems in the neck area.

If Botox is not appropriate for you, the first of two surgical options is what I call the **turkey gobbler release.** This involves making small incisions (3 mm) at the neck and cutting nick-like notches along the platysma bands. These small cuts serve to lessen the tension of the bands, thereby releasing pressure on the soft tissue of the neck. This procedure can be performed in a doctor's office with local anesthesia and the downtime following surgery is minimal. However, this procedure is effective only if the

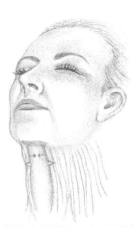

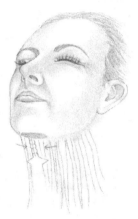

PLATYSMAPLASTY

A technique to tighten the separation of the platysma muscle that occurs with aging. A small incision is made under the chin, and the edges of the platysma muscles (platysmal bands) that have separated are brought back together in the midline, creating a smooth neck.

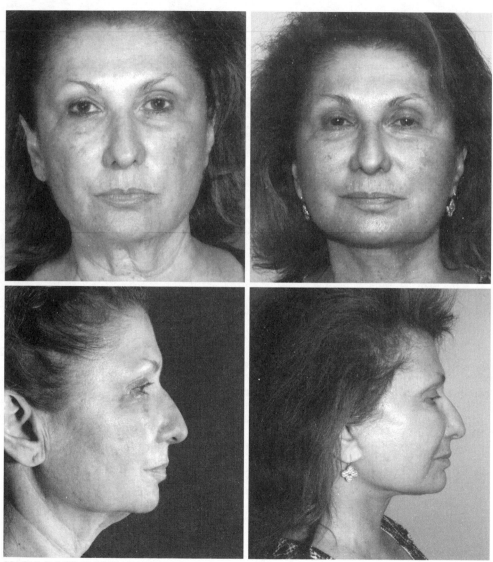

68-YEAR-OLD FEMALE WITH AN EXTENDED PLATYSMAPLASTY

platysma bands have just started to move and there is very little excess fat or skin. In my opinion, the turkey gobbler release produces better results than Botox—but not by a lot.

For patients with platysma bands that have widened enough to disrupt the soft tissue in their neck, a **corset procedure** (also called a platysmaplasty) is the best surgical option. A small incision is made just below the chin (where old childhood scars may already be present), and the platysmal split, which is located under the skin, is stitched together. Once that is done any minor problems relating to the soft tissue can be corrected with liposuction or skin redraping. If a large amount of excess skin remains, then more invasive procedures may be necessary. The skin can either be cut out directly under your neck or it can be pulled tighter with a facelift or an extended neck lift.

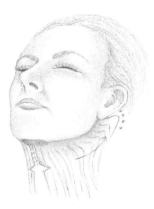

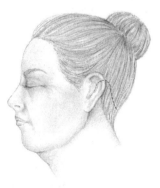

EXTENDED PLATYSMAPLASTY

A technique to tighten the platysma and neck structures while removing excess skin from behind the ears.

PROBLEM: EXCESS SKIN; SOLUTIONS: REDRAPING, RESECTION, AND FACELIFT

Excess skin ends up being a part of nearly every discussion relating to neck rejuvenation, and taking care of it properly is a critical element to successful results, no matter which primary surgical procedure you undergo. So when considering procedures to rejuvenate your neck it is important to familiarize yourself with the available options for dealing with excess skin.

The first, **skin redraping**, can be useful in making improvements to conformational wrinkles and is a good choice for someone who has some wrinkling in the neck area but does not have a lot of excess skin. Skin redraping corrects these wrinkles by lifting up the skin and letting it smooth itself out before being placed back in position. It's kind of like shaking out a wrinkled bedspread in the air and then laying it back down on the bed so it looks smoother. Redraping is different from a facelift in that it does not pull the skin at all or reattach it in a different place.

Another option—known medically as a **vertical submental skin excision**—cuts out the extra skin and is thus a good choice for those patients with a considerable amount of excess skin. This procedure can sometimes result in a slightly more noticeable scar under the chin, but since it is so effective in tightening up the neck area many patients feel it is worth it. Anecdotally, I have found that male patients who might be reluctant to undergo a full facelift opt for this procedure instead and have been very pleased with the results, despite the scar.

Finally, platysmal bands and excess neck skin can be treated with an **extended neck lift**. This procedure involves the platysmaplasty described above, along with a skin redraping and removal of excess skin behind the ears. Of course, for those interested in combining a neck lift with upper face lifting, a facelift can be done in conjunction with a neck procedure if the situation warrants it. Your doctor will weigh a variety of factors in determining what the proper course of action is. But keep in mind that sometimes it is easier to undergo more than one procedure simultaneously, thus combining recuperative periods and saving time in the long run.

You should note that any procedure dealing exclusively with excess skin (and not the underlying problem) is often a waste of time in the long run. Excess skin is usually symptomatic of other problems that need attention prior to redraping, resecting, or lifting being done. For example, in the case of widening platysma bands, even resecting a large amount of excess skin will not prevent the bands from widening further and creating the same problem again. Please be sure to keep this in mind when thinking about any type of neck rejuvenation.

The above procedures do entail some scarring. Skin redraping results in a small scar under your chin that is not particularly noticeable. A neck resection, which is used to get rid of larger amounts of excess skin, leaves a more visible vertical scar under your chin. Facelifts and neck lifts to address mild to moderate excess skin are usually done with an "S" scar behind the ear. Finally, facelifts dealing with large amounts of excess skin usually employ an omega scar that is located behind the ear on your scalp, concealed under your hair. The omega scar tends to be the choice among my more active patients because it allows them to wear their hair back in a ponytail with no visible signs of scarring.

THE CHIN

In plastic surgery, we make a distinction between surgery that is performed for rejuvenation purposes (to make you look younger) and surgery that is done for alteration purposes (to make you look different). Virtually all chin surgeries are done to alter the way you look and can be very successful in creating a more balanced face. Some people are just born with small chins, which can end up making other features on their face seem out of proportion. For example, a chin that lacks width and prominence can make your nose appear larger than it really is. Or a shorter-than-usual chin can change the shape and angle contours of your neck.

Chin implants are an effective way to correct this type of imbalance. A small incision is made either under the chin or inside the mouth and an implant of either silicone or polyethylene is placed on the bone at the subperiosteal plane. Both silicone and polyethylene implants are considered safe, but they do offer differing pros and cons. Polyethylene implants can feel more real, but they are less pliable, which makes them more difficult to insert and almost impossible to extract. Silicone implants are easier to insert and can be removed if necessary, but they can move around a bit once they have been implanted.

Surgeons can also change the shape of your chin by taking a piece of the chin bone and advancing it to a more prominent position before anchoring it in place with plates and screws. This procedure, called a horizontal osteotomy of the mandible (HOM), is more involved than implants because of a slightly higher risk of nerve injury as well as possible displacement of the muscles around the chin. In the end, an HOM usually offers a more natural result for a wider range of patients. In general, routine small chins are better treated with chin implants, while larger deformities or asymmetries are best treated with an HOM.

THE CHEEKS

Cheek implants can be used for the purpose of both rejuvenation and alteration. As I've mentioned, aging can lead to a "hollowed-out" appearance, especially around the cheek area due to loss of overall volume and fat. Cheek implants are very effective in creating a younger look by filling in that area of your face. They can be made of either silicone or polyethylene, offering patients the same pros and cons described above for chin implants. The surgery is performed by making an incision, either inside the mouth or under the eyelid, and the implants are placed on the subperiosteal plane in the cheek area.

If alteration is the goal, cheek implants are a relatively easy way to change the shape of a face. Adding volume to the midface creates a softer, cuter look. Placing the implants in a slightly different position will add width to a longer face, breaking up the lateral line and creating a more oval, aesthetically pleasing shape. Finally, cheek implants can be used to more clearly define the cheekbone. I still find it quite extraordinary how the overall balance and shape of a face can be improved just by using cheek implants. But, as with any procedure, serious consideration should be given to the benefits and risks of a surgery before proceeding.

WHAT TO EXPECT AFTER LOWER FACE SURGERY

Recovery times vary from procedure to procedure, so you will need to check with your doctor as to the amount of recuperative time your surgery requires. And while every plastic surgeon has his or her own list of postoperative "dos and don'ts" there are some general guidelines that are worth mentioning because they often lead to better results (and happier patients!). Just keep in mind that these are my particular recommendations and they may differ slightly from your surgeon's instructions.

- The patient should recover in a comfortable position, with the head elevated. It is important to have the back and shoulders supported with pillows as well.

- For the first 10 days, head movement should be minimal to avoid additional bruising and swelling. I advise my patients to imagine a pole running through their head, neck, and shoulders that, if it were real, would drastically limit their movement.

- Most physicians will prescribe cold compresses to be placed intermittently on the face for the first 24 hours after surgery. Be careful that these compresses are not too cold. In the early postoperative period overly cold compresses can cause frostbite, which ends up looking like a burn.

- An increase of blood pressure can lead to a facial hematoma. Therefore, patients must avoid any heavy lifting, excessive coughing or sneezing, bearing down while having a bowel movement, shouting, and absolutely all exercise. I once had a patient who went back to her daily sit-up regimen eight days after surgery because she felt so good. Unfortunately, the stress of the sit-ups raised her blood pressure and she developed a facial hematoma, prolonging her recovery.

• Salty foods cause you to retain water—which can add to your swelling—so they should be avoided for a few weeks after your operation.

Immediately following your surgery you will be quite incapacitated—to what degree will depend on the exact procedure you have undergone. I advise all of my patients to arrange for round-the-clock nursing during the first 24 hours in order to help with things like your positioning and taking the correct dosages of your medication. You can expect to awaken from surgery with a dressing that covers part or most of your face. Even though this can feel claustrophobic it is there for a reason: to minimize swelling and the risk of bleeding. Therefore your dressings must be kept in place. Many surgeons now use drains (tubes designed to get rid of excess fluid, blood, and serum under the skin) as they help speed the healing process. These drains are typically removed after two days and the sutures are usually removed after five days, just as the swelling starts to recede. By the tenth day the bruising should be almost if not entirely gone and patients can typically return to their normal routine.

I have found that my patients are often eager to wash their hair as soon as the immediate discomfort of the surgery wears off. This is a good thing as it provides a psychological boost and helps maintain overall hygiene near the traumatized area. I advise my patients to use Johnson's No More Tangles Shampoo + Conditioner—it is gentle but effective in washing away any dried blood remaining on the scalp.

COST OF THE PROCEDURE

Fees for any of the above procedures will vary widely based on the surgeon's experience, the geographic location of the facility, and the specific parameters of each procedure. So the following figures should be considered a very loose guide as to what to expect. You will need to do research in your area to get a more accurate idea of the total cost.

When calculating the potential costs, you should be aware that your financial commitment is often broken down into three separate components: the anesthesiologist, the facility, and the surgeon. The anesthesia fee is usually about $600 for the first 30 minutes in the operating room, with each additional 30-minute block charged at a rate of $300. Facility fees will vary and can be either a flat rate or an itemized bill. If possible, always try to negotiate a fixed flat fee that is all-inclusive. That way, you won't be surprised by any added charges you are not prepared to absorb. On average, the facility fee for a same-day discharge is approximately $1,800 to $3,000. Finally, plastic surgeon fees will vary widely based on their experience, which is reflected in the ranges below.

Procedure	Cost[†]
Facelift	$7,500–12,000
Neck lift	$5,000–8,000
Chin implants	$2,500–5,000
Cheek implants	$2,500–4,000

[†]Note: All prices are in U.S. dollars, current as of 2009.

LOWER FACE SELF-ASSESSMENT

Before making an appointment for an initial consultation with a plastic surgeon, it might be useful to perform a few quick tests on yourself in front of a mirror. Obviously, a plastic surgeon will assess your needs in a more medically sound manner! But now that you understand your facial anatomy, as well as your varied options for rejuvenation, it cannot hurt to spend a few minutes getting a sense of how plastic surgery might improve your overall appearance.

Looking in the mirror, take note of the border of your jawline, your marionette lines, and the position of your cheek. Give a big smile and place a finger on the highest point of your cheek, holding the soft tissue in its new position. Then relax your face again. If you see a dramatic change in the jawline, marionette lines, or cheek fullness your SMAS has started to sag and you would probably benefit from a facelift.

Now pinch the skin in your neck area. Is there more than half an inch of tissue between your fingers? If so, then you may need to have fat removed. Next, stare in the mirror and use your neck muscles (platysma) to pull down your lower lip so your lower teeth are revealed. If you see vertical lines extending from your chin down your neck while holding this position you may need a platysmaplasty. Finally, pull the skin of your neck toward your ears on both sides. If you see a significant improvement then you may benefit from a neck lift.

Chapter 7

UPPER FACE, EYES, AND BROW

"The absence of flaw in beauty is itself a flaw."

—Havelock Ellis

M ost people think of the eyes as the window to the soul. While that may or may not be true, they are undoubtedly the focal point of your face. As you grow older, the pull of gravity and loss of elasticity in the eye area become harder to ignore. Upper face rejuvenation refers to a wide variety of procedures used to correct signs of aging to your eyes, eyebrows, and forehead. When done properly, these procedures can provide you with not only exceptional results but also the most bang for your buck, precisely because the area is the focal point of your face. If a patient comes to me not quite ready to have a facelift but wanting to look younger, the eye area is usually the first place we discuss.

This chapter will help you understand the basic anatomy of your upper face, how age affects those elements, and what your surgical and nonsurgical options are. Again, once you have educated yourself about the available rejuvenating procedures it will be easier for you to meet with your doctor and sort through what may or may not be right for you.

ANATOMY AND THE EFFECTS OF AGING

The five anatomical elements most critical to the overall appearance of your upper face are the skin, muscle, hair, eyebrows/forehead, and eyes. Since general facial anatomy was covered in the previous chapter, I will keep this discussion specific to the eye and forehead area.

SKIN

While all of your skin ages in much the same way, the skin of your upper face is slightly different in that it is home to some of the thickest and thinnest skin on your body. Your forehead, which has very thick skin, is prone to a high concentration of dynamic wrinkles from years of communicating emotion. It is also where frown lines appear (also referred to as "11s") when the eyebrows are pulled toward the center to show displeasure. And the very thin skin at the outside corner of your eyes develops wrinkles—crow's-feet—from decades of smiling and squinting.

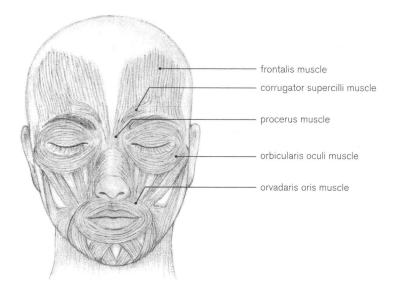

FACIAL MUSCLES (WITH SKIN CUT AWAY)

The corrugator supercilli muscle contracts to make frown lines. The procerus muscle contracts to create the wrinkle on the top of the nose. The orbicularis oculi muscle contracts to create crow's-feet. The orvadaris oris muscle contracts to make the vertical lines around the mouth.

MUSCLE

There are four muscles of most concern to plastic surgeons working on this area of your face—the frontalis, the corrugator supercilli, the procerus, and the orbicularis oculi of each eye. While I don't want to overwhelm you with too many medical terms, these four are critical to the way your upper face ages, so you will find it helpful to know about them.

- **The frontalis muscle** is located in the central two-thirds of your forehead. This muscle is responsible for lifting your eyebrows to communicate surprise as well as to keep the skin of your upper lid in place as it becomes heavier. To understand how this muscle works, elevate your eyebrows as high as you can—you will feel your upper eyelids become lighter and more open. In general, muscles lengthen as you age, and the frontalis is no exception. However, there is a particularly curious phenomenon that occurs in this area. As the skin and muscle of the eyebrow start to sag, your brain transmits signals to the frontalis muscle to work harder to lift the heavier eyebrow skin to keep it from weighing on the very thin skin of your upper eyelid—which it does. But, while the problem of a sagging eyebrow may be corrected, the end result is the creation of new dynamic wrinkles from the frontalis muscle working overtime! These are the horizontal wrinkles of the forehead. Thus, some forehead wrinkles are due to sagging skin of the eyelids and eyebrow, and not the forehead.

- Two muscles, the **corrugator supercilli** and the **procerus**, form a "W" across your forehead and are key in helping you to communicate emotion through facial expression. The corrugator supercilli pulls each eyebrow toward the center, creating the vertical frown lines, and the procerus muscle pulls the skin above the nose downward, creating a horizontal crease above the nose. So while these muscles are useful in letting people know you are not happy, they also create grooves in your skin from years of doing so. The good news is that since that is all these muscles do, they are nonessential and thus can be injected with Botox to paralyze them or they can be surgically removed (more on that later).

- Around each eye is a circular muscle that begins and ends in the same place, the **orbicularis oculi** muscle. In addition to holding your eye in its socket, this muscle allows you to squint and blink. To understand how a circular muscle affects your skin when it contracts, think of a soft pouch with a drawstring. When you close the pouch by pulling the string, the material folds over itself and wrinkles. The same is true when the orbicularis oculi is contracted—the skin around your eye gets pulled tighter, which creates crow's-feet as you age.

HAIR

While I cover general information about hair in chapter 11, in this section it is important to mention that as you age your hair—and hairline—can change, affecting the overall appearance of your upper face. A receding hairline can make you look older by altering the symmetry of your face, usually by elongating it. In addition, your hairline becomes particularly important when considering which type of upper face rejuvenation is right for you. If you already have a high hairline, or one that is rising with age, your plastic surgeon should be very careful to avoid any procedure that could raise your hairline any further.

EYEBROWS AND FOREHEAD

In any discussion of upper face rejuvenation, the eyebrows and forehead are considered one unit. Thus, the term *brow lift* really refers to a surgical enhancement done to both the eyebrow and the forehead. Remember that the frontalis muscle of the forehead holds your eyebrows in place, so the two areas are quite literally connected, which is why it would make no medical sense to approach them separately. As you age, your eyebrows will sag due to gravity as well as a lengthening of the frontalis muscle and forehead skin. This changing position of your eyebrow in relation to your forehead and hairline must be taken into consideration when weighing your options for rejuvenating procedures in this area. For example, a brow lift should never position the inner two-thirds of your eyebrow (that section closest to the bridge of your nose) above the orbital rim (the edge of the bone that surrounds your eye), or it will give you an unnatural surprised look. Finally, as you age your forehead is prone to dynamic wrinkles from years of frowning or worrying.

EYES

When considering possible surgical procedures, the eye area should be approached with care because this whole area is quite delicate. The upper and lower sections are considered separately and handled in different ways. The upper lid presents problems of excess or sagging skin and some bulging fat; the lower lid is plagued by bulges of fat, a weakening of the muscles that hold the eyelid up, and deepening grooves below the eyelid made by the soft tissue of your cheek being pulled down by gravity.

CHOOSING UPPER FACE PROCEDURES

Now that you understand how aging affects the anatomy of your upper face, it will be easier to decide which surgical and nonsurgical procedures are appropriate for you. The four main upper face aging issues are sagging eyebrows, forehead wrinkles, upper lid problems, and lower lid problems. Looking at the chart on the next page, you can see that no single procedure is designed to tackle all of these at the same time. You will also note that though some procedures are tailor-made for one problem they can be wholly inappropriate for others, so it is critical to have a specific understanding about what you are tackling and how to achieve the best possible results.

Age-related Problem	Anatomic Problem	Corrective Procedures
sagging eyebrows	excess forehead skin, sagging frontalis muscle	forehead/brow lift, browpexy
forehead wrinkles	excess forehead skin, sagging eyebrows, excess upper eyelid skin, sagging frontalis muscle	forehead/brow lift
upper eyelid puffiness	excess eyelid skin, herniated eyelid fat, sagging eyebrows	upper eyelid blepharoplasty, brow lift
lower eyelid puffiness/bags	herniated eyelid fat, sagging muscle	lower eyelid blepharoplasty
lower eyelid sagging (bloodhound look)	weakening of the lower eyelid muscles and ligaments, midface sagging	lower eyelid tightening procedures, midface lift

BOTOX

Because wrinkles appear on your forehead due to dynamic changes caused by muscles used to communicate emotion, it follows logically that if those muscles were rendered unable to contract, the wrinkles would go away. That is exactly how Botox works. Small doses of Botox—which is a protein produced by the bacteria *Clostridium botulinum*—are injected into your forehead, which basically paralyzes the area that has been injected. The forehead is the only place this can be done because the muscles there have no other job than to control facial expression.

While most patients undergo Botox treatments in order to get rid of forehead wrinkles, it can also be used as a temporary, nonsurgical brow lift. Remember that with age the heavier skin of your eyebrow starts to sag into the very delicate eyelid area and your brain sends a signal to the frontalis muscle to lift that skin up. If Botox is injected into the area close to the inner two-thirds of the eyebrow, then the only part of the frontalis muscle still able to respond to the brain to lift the heavier skin is the outer edge (about 1 cm on either side), which has not been injected. This nonparalyzed section of the frontalis muscle lifts the outer third of your eyebrow—giving you a nonsurgical brow lift.

As with anything, the use of Botox has its own distinct set of pros and cons. The upsides are that it is nonsurgical, is safe, and requires virtually no downtime. Mitigating these benefits is the fact that Botox is temporary, lasting no more than six months. I also find that a Botox brow lift can make people look a little peaky, as if they are in a state of perpetual surprise—something a good surgical procedure would avoid.

FILLERS

There are four areas of your upper face that can, to varying degrees, benefit from the use of fillers—crow's-feet, nasojugal grooves (the tear trough), corrugator lines, and frown lines. Before discussing these specific areas, I will review some of the general information on fillers that was covered in chapter 3.

Plastic surgeons use three types of fillers—temporary, permanent, and your own fat—to smooth out areas of your facial skin that have developed wrinkles or grooves with age. Although fillers can be effective on their own, they are often used in conjunction with other procedures (such as Botox) to enhance the end result.

As I have stated before, I do not use any permanent fillers on my patients. There are a number of reasons why, primary among them is that they do not age with your face and they are impossible to take out. So if the filler starts to look out of place as your facial anatomy changes, there is nothing a surgeon can do.

Crow's-feet. These small wrinkles at the outer edge of your eye present a challenge because the skin is very delicate in this area and the muscle is strong. Thus, after a filler is injected and the muscle continues to work, the filler can be pushed to either side. This often results in a deepening of the crease—exactly the opposite of what was intended! Fillers can also leave bumps in the area because of the thinness of the skin. It is not uncommon to actually see the filler under the thin skin as a bluish hue. It is for all of these reasons that I highly recommend using Botox instead of fillers for crow's-feet.

Nasojugal Grooves. Also known as the tear trough, these deep creases under your eye can be rejuvenated particularly well with the use of fillers. The various soft tissues near your eye are located on different planes of your face and, as you age, these tissues can shift and collide, creating a deep groove. An easy way to think of this is a crack made in the Earth's surface after an earthquake. Of course, the actual movement of fat and soft tissue under your skin is slower and not nearly as dramatic, but the end result is similar—a "crack" at the surface that needs to be repaired.

When working to correct nasojugal grooves my filler of choice is a patient's fat. I find that not only does it last longer and age with the patient in a more natural way, but it also offers a less costly alternative to Restylane or Juvéderm. Due to the depth of the nasojugal grooves, the procedure often requires a considerable amount of filler—up to 4 or 5 cc per groove. When using Restylane or Juvéderm, a single treatment with that much filler can run close to $5,000—a cost that can quickly become prohibitive when considering that these treatments are temporary. Fat fillers are often temporary as well, but there is the chance that it can last for many years in some cases, and there is no increased expense for using larger amounts. For example, if I am harvesting a patient's fat, the cost will be the same whether I take out 1 cc or 10 cc. With manufactured temporary fillers you are paying for each drop you use, which is why in areas that require large amounts, like the nasojugal grooves, the cost becomes a serious consideration.

Corrugator and Frown Lines. Fillers can be used in these areas, but since they are temporary, like Botox, it is just as easy to paralyze the muscle causing the lines, rather than filling in the grooves. In addition, with Botox you do not run the risk of a filler shifting position, as can sometimes happen when correcting for dynamic changes.

BROW LIFTS

According to generally accepted ideals of beauty, a woman's eyebrow should have a slight arch at the outer third of the eye and the inner part of the eyebrow should be positioned at the orbital rim or below it. For men, the eyebrow should be completely horizontal on the face, but it, too, should be positioned no higher than the orbital rim.

During any procedure done in the eyebrow and forehead area—whether it be to lift sagging skin or to get rid of wrinkles—a plastic surgeon has to be careful not to over-correct, leaving you with a less-than-ideal shape or position of your eyebrow. Another challenge of working in this area is making sure not to disrupt the symmetry of your face, especially that all-important relative space between your eyebrow and hairline. In fact, your existing hairline will be the most important factor in determining what can—and cannot—be done here.

Deciding which brow lift procedure is right for you will depend on which part of the eyebrow/forehead is going to be corrected, if excess skin has to be removed, where the scars need to be located, and the length of recovery time.

Endoscopic Brow Lift. This relatively new procedure, which is the least invasive of the four options, offers patients the benefits of a brow lift but with a shorter recovery time. The surgeon makes five small incisions at your hairline and, using an endoscope, works below the soft tissue (close to the bone) to pull everything up toward the hair-line. The soft tissue—which includes your skin, fat, muscle, and fascia—is then held in place by tiny screws that have been drilled into the bone. In addition to less downtime, there are a couple of benefits to an endoscopic brow lift. Since the surgeon is working in a deep plane, the risk of nerve damage is almost nonexistent. And because an endoscope is used, the scars will be quite small.

As for downsides, this brow lift can change a patient's hairline to varying degrees—how much so will depend, in large part, on the "before" hairline. Also, an endoscopic brow lift does not get rid of extra skin—nothing is being cut out—so the original problems of excessively loose or saggy skin can eventually reappear. Thus, while this option is less invasive, it also tends to be less durable than the other three brow lifts, which actually resect skin. Some of you may be wondering why pulling many layers

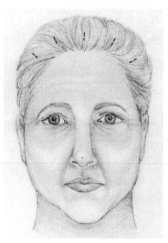

ENDOSCOPIC BROW LIFT

Five small incisions are made within the hairline. The skin and soft tissue are separated from the underlying structures and then lifted upward. The hairline is elevated as a result of this technique.

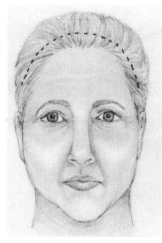

CORONAL BROW LIFT

A single long incision is made across the scalp from ear to ear, 1 inch (2–3 cm) behind the hairline. Some surgeons will make the incision zigzag to better camouflage the scar. The hairline is elevated in this technique.

of tissue at the same time can offer noticeable results in an endoscopic brow lift but not in a deep plane or subperiosteal facelift (described in chapter 6). This is due, in large part, to the fact that the individual layers of tissue in this area are more adherent to each other, thus minimizing the need to pull really hard in order to achieve optimum results.

Coronal Brow Lift. Of the four brow lift options, this procedure has been around the longest. An ear-to-ear incision is made about 1 inch (2–3 cm) behind the hairline, the soft tissue of the forehead and eyebrow area is pulled up, any extra skin is cut away, and then the skin is reattached to the scalp at the incision. There are two obvious benefits to this procedure: The scar is hidden behind the hairline and the results are durable because skin is being excised. The downsides are that the hairline must be raised when the skin is reattached (since the surgeon is cutting behind the hairline) and there can be nerve loss because the incision for this procedure is large and can potentially do damage to the many nerve fibers in the area. The coronal brow lift is not for everyone, but it is a good option for patients who need to have a lot of skin excised and who can afford to have their hairline raised slightly.

Lateral Brow Lift. This brow lift works on the outer third of the forehead and eyebrow—the area where there is no muscle (remember, the frontalis, corrugator, and procerus are all located in the middle of your forehead). It is because this area is without muscle that it is more prone to the pull of gravity and is often the first—or only—part of the brow to sag. Surgeons can perform a lateral brow lift with or without an endoscope assist (the length of the scar will depend on whether one is used or not). There is often excess tissue created by this lateral pull and it should be cut out during the brow lift to ensure longer-lasting results. The main benefit of a lateral brow lift is that there is no danger of changing your hairline since the surgeon is pulling tissue up into the area where the height of the hairline includes the sideburn. This can be a very important consideration if you already have a high hairline and do not want to risk further raising it in surgery.

Pretrichial Brow Lift. This procedure is identical to the coronal brow lift except that the ear-to-ear incision is made at the hairline rather than 1 inch (2–3 cm) behind it. The main reason for a patient choosing this brow lift is that it allows for a considerable amount of excess skin to be cut out while not raising the hairline. Of course, the problem with this incision is that it leaves a visible scar. Sometimes it may be necessary to use hair transplants to hide the scar. Like the coronal and lateral brow lifts, this procedure offers patients lasting results because skin is being excised.

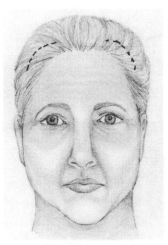

LATERAL BROW LIFT

Two lateral incisions minimize scarring and loss of sensation to the scalp. The lift for this technique centers over the outer eyebrow and eyelids. The hairline is not elevated with this technique.

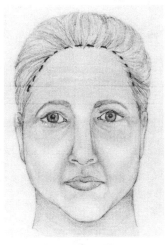

PRETRICHIAL BROW LIFT

A single incision at the hairline is used for patients with a high hairline at the outset. This allows for elevating the brow, removing excess forehead skin, and no hairline changes. A drawback to this technique is the potential for visible scarring.

Brow Lift Technique	Incision	Degree of improvement	Hair Loss	Hairline Changes	Sensory Loss
endoscopic	5 small incisions in the hairline	+	minimal	elevates hairline	minimal
coronal	large incision in hairline from ear to ear	++++	can be significant	elevates hairline	with all patients
lateral	two small incisions in the hair in the temple region	limited to outer portion of the forehead and eyebrows	moderate to minimal	no elevation	only behind small incisions
pretrichial	at the hairline, can be visible	++++	no hair loss	no elevation	with all patients

BLEPHAROPLASTY

Your eyes are affected by aging in a variety of ways. As mentioned earlier, plastic surgeons divide the eye area into two distinct sections—upper and lower. This is done not only because the problems tend to be slightly different between the two but also because the lower eye area can be quite tricky to work on. Thus, I would strongly advise that if you need a lower blepharoplasty—especially one that requires dealing with the muscle—you consult a plastic surgeon who has made the lower eyelid their specialty.

Upper Blepharoplasty. Depending on the situation, an upper blepharoplasty can entail excising saggy skin, removing the weak muscle, getting rid of herniated fat, or any combination thereof. An incision is made below what plastic surgeons call the "transition skin" (the area between your eyebrow and your eyelid) and any excised skin is taken from the eyelid—not the transition area. The removal of any fat or muscle is also done through this incision. The main caution to be aware of when considering any surgical procedure to the upper eyelid is taking too much skin out. This can either leave an ugly scar in the transition zone or, worse, affect your ability to close your eyelid.

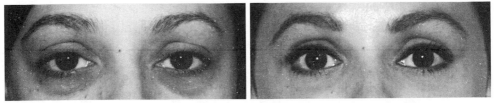

32-YEAR-OLD WITH LOWER LID BAGS AND DISCOLORATION

A transconjunctival lower blepharoplasty was performed and the area was treated with hydroquinone.

Sometimes a brow lift needs to be done in conjunction with an upper blepharoplasty in order to avoid the temptation of trying to accomplish too much while only working on the upper lid. Remember that a surgeon can always take more out but can never put back what has been excised.

An upper eyelid incision can also be used to remove the corrugator supercilli muscle (minimizing frown lines) or to perform a minimal lift of the eyebrow called a browpexy. Using this incision for a limited eyebrow lift is a particularly strong option for men because it avoids scarring to the forehead, where eventual baldness could reveal a previously concealed scar.

Lower Blepharoplasty. The most common lower eyelid problems that occur with aging are crepey skin and herniated fat. But before reviewing the three procedures available to address these issues, it is important to understand the particular risks associated with working in the lower eyelid area. Proper movement of the lower eyelid is critical to healthy eye function—most especially with regard to keeping your eyes hydrated. If, after surgery, the lower eyelid does not sit on your eyeball correctly, the tears and lubrication made by the lacrimal gland will not function properly. This can cause dry eye, which is terribly uncomfortable to live with.

Furthering the challenge of the area is that the muscle of the lower eyelid is somewhat of an anomaly. Muscles usually flex in the direction of the desired movement. For example, the upper eyelid muscles pull upward when it opens. But since the lower eyelid muscle is perpendicular to the direction it needs to move in (it is stretched

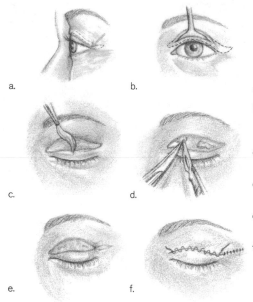

a.

b.

c.

d.

e.

f.

a. Excess skin is marked for excision.

b. The amount of excision is checked by a pinch test to ensure that the proper amount of tissue is being removed.

c. Excess skin and muscle are removed according to the markings previously performed.

d. Excess fat is easily and safely removed. If too much fat is removed, a hollowed-out appearance will result.

e. A stay stitch is applied to ensure that the skin edges close nicely.

f. The eyelid is closed with fine stitches that allow for an almost imperceptible scar inside the eyelid crease.

UPPER BLEPHAROPLASTY

horizontally across the lower eyelid even though the movement is vertical) this area is anatomically complicated and needs to be handled with great care. If a surgeon were to inadvertently damage the muscle that controls the movement of the lower eyelid or weaken the ligaments that hold the lower lid intact, your eye could suffer long-term damage and start to sag, giving you the appearance of a bloodhound—not quite the desired result of the surgery. I will reiterate that the lower lid blepharoplasty requires extreme care in its execution and should be performed only by experts in the field.

In a **skin-only lower blepharoplasty**, the skin and muscle have to be carefully separated before the skin can be excised. This procedure is a good option for people who have crepey skin under their eyes rather than big bags due to herniated fat being pushed out of the orbital rim. The incision for this procedure is made just under the eyelashes and is difficult—if not impossible—to see. This technique is rather straightforward with little risk of doing long-term damage to the muscle of the eye. The only limitation is that it is good for the skin only.

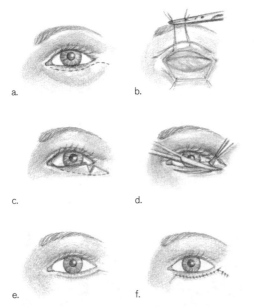

a. A mark is placed in the location for the planned incision just under the eyelashes and extending past the corner of the eye in a natural skin crease.

b. An incision is made under the lower eyelid skin and muscle as per the previous markings. Any excess fat is removed.

c. The amount of excess skin to be removed is determined by gently lifting the skin and marking with a cut the excess amount. More than any other excision, overexcision in this step can be disastrous for the patient, resulting in the lower lid being pulled down.

d. After double-checking the proper amount of skin to be excised, the excess is removed.

e. At this point the skin should be brought together with minimal tension and without any effort.

f. Finally, without tension the incision is closed. A properly executed lower blepharoplasty will leave some fine wrinkles in the lower lid.

LOWER BLEPHAROPLASTY (SKIN/MUSCLE TECHNIQUE)

A **skin and muscle lower blepharoplasty** is fraught with risk because the actual eyelid muscle is being worked on. This technique is used to remove excess skin and muscle, as well as remove the bulging fat that creates the lower eyelid bags. The incision is similar to that of the skin-only lower blepharoplasty but is made through the muscle as well. Some skin is taken out, but the primary objective of this procedure is to get the muscle repositioned back to where it should be and stitched in place.

The last option, a **transconjunctival lower blepharoplasty**, is a good choice for someone who has a lot of excess fat creating a bulge in the lower eyelid. This is the safest of the three options because the surgeon doesn't go near the muscle. A small incision is made inside the eyelid, which allows for easy access to the fat. Once the fat is removed there isn't even a need for stitches—this area heals nicely on its own. Very often excess skin becomes a problem after the procedure and there are three options for dealing with this issue. A skin-only blepharoplasty can be done to excise the tissue. This combination of procedures allows for removing the fat from behind the muscle and the skin from in front of the muscle while never actually touching the orbicularis oculi—a safe way to accomplish great results in the lower eyelid area. Alternatively, the excess skin can be tightened up with a laser or chemical peel. I avoid both of these because the downtime is longer and the risks more significant than simply excising the extra skin.

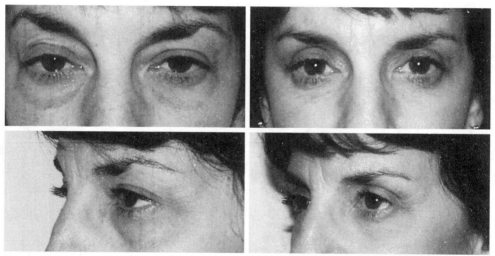

56-YEAR-OLD FEMALE WITH EXCESS UPPER AND LOWER EYELID SKIN, FAT, AND EYEBROW SAGGING

An upper and lower (skin/muscle) blepharoplasty with a lateral brow lift was performed. Note: The eyebrows are in a more relaxed position after the brow lift. Prior to the procedure, the excess tissue caused extra weight on the upper eyelid, which was relieved by excessive unnatural lifting of the eyebrow.

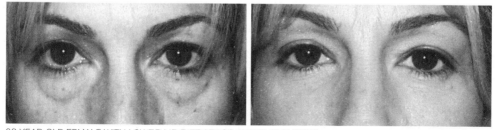

38-YEAR-OLD FEMALE WITH LOWER LID FATTY BAGS AND FLAT CHEEKS

A transconjunctival lower blepharoplasty (for removal of the bags) with autologous fat grafts to the cheek was performed.

Chapter 8

NOSE

"I was going to have cosmetic surgery until I noticed that the doctor's office was full of portraits by Picasso."

—Rita Rudner

Your nose—even if it is perfectly shaped—is the most prominent and noticeable feature of your face. Thus it would follow that if your nose is not perfect it becomes quite hard to ignore. The good news is that there are myriad and subtle changes that a surgeon can make to correct these imperfections, giving you the nose that is truly right for you.

Before I discuss what makes a nose right for your face, it is important to point out two caveats as you consider rhinoplasty. First, this area of your anatomy is critical to your health—after all, you breathe through your nose. Therefore, the first rule of any rhinoplasty must be "do no harm." A bad nose job can affect your breathing for the rest of your life, so the importance of a safe and appropriate surgery cannot be overemphasized. Second, because of the nose's anatomical complexity, you should only consider a surgeon who specializes in this area. We have all seen the horror photos in the tabloids of nose jobs gone bad, and often those procedures were performed by surgeons who did not have the requisite experience to execute the procedure properly. So it is extremely important to choose a surgeon who has a proven mastery over the techniques necessary to solve your specific problems.

In addition to finding the right doctor, your chance of a successful procedure will be greatly enhanced if you take the time to learn the basic anatomy of your nose as well as to familiarize yourself with the three procedures used to correct most problems. Then you will be able to ask the pertinent questions during your consultation, ensuring that you go into your procedure with realistic expectations and a high comfort level about what is happening.

Up to 15 percent of all rhinoplasties end up being redone. Sometimes these second-time corrections are unavoidable, but more often than not they are due to surgical inexperience. And since a secondary rhinoplasty is always going to be more complicated than the first, it is best to get it right the first time!

NOSE SHAPE: ETHNICITY AND BALANCE

Once you have found a surgeon who specializes in rhinoplasty surgery, you will need to be ready to tackle the question of what shape nose will enhance your face. While that decision will ultimately be very personal, it is dictated in large part by cultural and ethnic norms along with your anatomy. Even in today's world of political correctness, cultural norms of what people "should" look like in relation to their ethnicity are hard to ignore.

I often have patients come to me with a photograph of an actress or actor, point to it and say, "I want that nose." And while it may be anatomically possible to make those changes, it might not be the right nose for this particular patient. The vast majority of nose surgeries are altering (rather than rejuvenating), which means that patients who are considering a rhinoplasty are doing so because they want to change the way they look. With rhinoplasties this usually involves correcting the nose so it draws less attention, whether by straightening, narrowing, shortening, or lengthening it. A surgeon should never consider reshaping a nose in a way that does not fit into cultural or ethnic norms. That would only end up drawing *more* attention—the exact opposite of the desired effect.

I once had a patient from Rome who taught me a thing or two about cultural norms. She came to see me about correcting a wide nasal tip, but during her preliminary exam I noticed that she also had a mild bump on her nasal profile. When I mentioned that I could fix the bump as well, you would have thought I told her I didn't like pasta! She explained to me in no uncertain terms that a bump on the nose in Italy is considered beautiful and she did not want me to go near it. I learned a valuable lesson that day: cultural norms do endure and are an important part of any successful rhinoplasty.

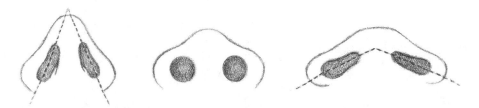

NOSTRIL SHAPES AND THEIR ETHNICITY
The axis of the nostril changes with ethnicity. A Caucasian nostril is pointy (left). The Asian nostril is rounder (center). The black nose is longer and flatter (right).

Cultural norms are most often determined by anatomical characteristics. For example, the majority of Asians and blacks have wider noses than those of Caucasians. If an Asian woman were to come to me asking for a small, pixie-type nose I would explain the challenges—both technically as well as culturally—of such a procedure. Keep in mind there are ways a good surgeon can subtly reshape a nose to make it fit better on your face, enhancing your appearance while remaining true to cultural expectations. But to do a complete overhaul, with the goal of changing an ethnic look—even if it can be done safely—very often ends in disappointment. And, quite frankly, an extreme change like that usually cannot be safely performed. One just has to think of the late pop star whose nose was fodder for late-night comics to understand the point I am trying to make. Not only did his nose look out of place on his face, but the extreme surgeries that were required to achieve that shape destroyed his nose.

It is also important that your nose properly balance your face. And this is where a good surgeon becomes important. Everyone's face is unique, and it will be up to your doctor to determine the finely calibrated changes needed to achieve the right look. More so than in any other facial surgery, there is pure artistry involved in a successful rhinoplasty. A properly balanced look can only be achieved by approaching the face as a whole and understanding how the problems in the nose area are affecting the rest of your facial features. For example, a narrow nose can make your cheeks look wider from the front. A longer nose, viewed from the side, will make your chin appear smaller. These secondary problems—wider cheeks or a smaller chin—are really just optical illusions and will disappear after a successful rhinoplasty. So it is important to remember to always view your nose in relation to your whole face.

Most nose jobs are performed on people simply looking to change the noses they were born with—the most common complaints being bumps on the nose and wide or distorted nasal tips. Other rhinoplasties are done to correct damage caused by trauma, returning a nose to as close to its original shape as possible. Aging can affect your nose, as well, so some rhinoplasties are performed for rejuvenating purposes. Whatever reason you may have for considering a rhinoplasty, before you even speak to a surgeon you should acquire a basic understanding of your nasal anatomy.

NASAL ANATOMY

Each specific area of your nose has a name. It is a good idea to familiarize yourself with these terms before consulting a doctor about a rhinoplasty to make it easier to communicate exactly which areas you consider problematic.

As a starting point take a step back—way back to your high school biology class. More than likely there was a skeleton in the corner of the lab collecting dust. If you think about it you will probably remember that the skeleton did not have a nose. That

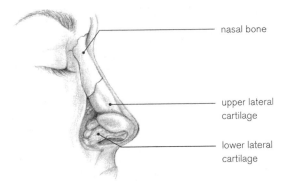

nasal bone

upper lateral cartilage

lower lateral cartilage

INTERNAL NASAL ANATOMY (SIDE VIEW)

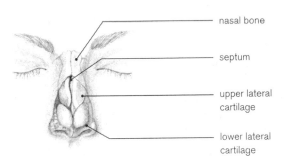

nasal bone

septum

upper lateral cartilage

lower lateral cartilage

INTERNAL NASAL ANATOMY (FRONTAL VIEW)

The upper third of the nose is comprised of nasal bones. The middle third of the nose is comprised of the upper lateral cartilage on either side of a rigid support called the septum. The lower third of the nose is comprised of the lower cartilage; the inner part of this structure (medial crura) makes up the columella, and the lateral part of this structure makes up the majority of the nasal tip and nostril rim.

is because a large portion of your nose is made of cartilage, not bone. This fact alone has much to do with why rhinoplasties are so challenging—both to get them right the first time and to fix them the second time.

Cartilage is difficult to work with for many reasons, primary among them that it has what doctors call "memory." This means that even when adjustments are made, the natural impulse is for your nose cartilage to spring back to its original position. There are surgical techniques that can be used to thwart this movement, but sometimes the techniques themselves can cause problems. For example, a surgeon can make very fine cuts to release the forces that are distorting the cartilage, thus allowing it to move in the desired direction. Unfortunately these cuts can cause scar tissue, which might result in a contraction that encourages the cartilage to return to its previously distorted position. In addition, scar tissue can reduce blood supply to the cartilage, which has the effect of diminishing its structural integrity. Once this happens the cartilage can start to collapse, creating problems with the patient's breathing (remember our late pop star?). There are many other possible pitfalls when surgically manipulating cartilage—too many to list here—but the above examples should serve to illustrate my point that this area is delicate and should be handled by a specialist.

Roughly speaking, the upper one-third of your nose is bone, while the lower two-thirds is comprised of cartilage. It follows that since bone is easier to manipulate than cartilage, a rhinoplasty becomes more complex as the area to be worked on moves down the nose. This means a fix to the upper-third of your nose is less complicated and has a higher success rate than a rhinoplasty performed on the lower third, where there is no bone at all.

The anatomical elements that relate most directly to the aesthetics of the nose (those parts of the nose we can see from the outside) are the glabella, the midvault, the nasal tip, the columella, and the alar base. These five terms and their corresponding

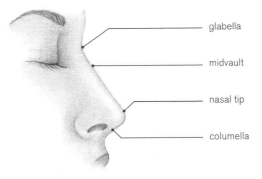

glabella

midvault

nasal tip

columella

NASAL LANDMARKS (SIDE VIEW)

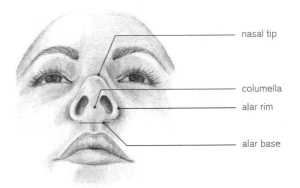

nasal tip

columella

alar rim

alar base

NASAL LANDMARKS (FRONTAL VIEW)

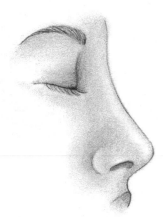

PROFILE OF NOSE
WITHOUT GLABELLA

The lack of a glabella makes the nose
appear longer than a similar length nose.

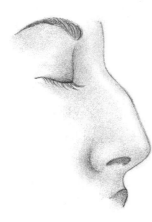

NASAL PROFILE WITH A
DORSAL HUMP (MIDVAULT)

areas will be the most important for you to have a grasp of when discussing your nose with a doctor.

GLABELLA

The glabella is the area at the top of your nose between your eyebrows. This area should be recessed in order to create a properly balanced look. If it is straight—with no indentation—then there will be no visual break between your forehead and your nose. Without that small dip to make the delineation, your nose tends to look as if it were an extension of your forehead, appearing longer than it actually is. Sometimes if a person does not have a recessed glabella but has a bump on her nose a visual break is achieved anyway. Keep in mind, however, that if a rhinoplasty gets rid of the bump, the lack of a recessed glabella will suddenly elongate the nose. More so than any other area of your face, the aesthetics of your nose is all about how the separate parts of the whole relate to each other. Therefore, when you change one thing the appearance of all else will shift, if even slightly.

MIDVAULT

As the name implies, this area is the middle third of your nose and is comprised mainly of cartilage, with some bone at the top edge. The septum, which is cartilage that separates the right and left nasal airways, moves downward from the nasal bones in the midline and extends toward the nasal tip. The upper lateral cartilages are anchored to the septum and flare out toward each cheek to add support to the skin. Both the septum and the upper lateral cartilage are very important to your breathing function—and thus a tricky area to work on.

You have probably heard of a deviated septum if you watch a lot of ESPN, but you don't need to be hit in the nose with a fist or a hockey puck to have one—it can be a genetic condition as well. Whatever the cause, a deviated septum means the cartilage in this area has become twisted. The outward sign of this condition tends to be a nose that looks bent, collapsed, or otherwise not straight in the midvault region. And while that might be unattractive, the true downside of a deviated septum is internal, as it disrupts your breathing and affects your ability to properly filter the air you draw in through your nose. Turbinates, which act as your body's air purifiers and humidifiers, are located in each airway. A deviated septum can cause the turbinates to swell, which may have the unfortunate effect of forcing you to breathe through your mouth—which performs no purifying function at all. There is no need to panic if you have been told you have a slightly deviated septum, however. The above problems present themselves only when the septum is seriously out of position.

NASAL TIP

Even though the tip represents the smallest third of your nose, it actually determines a large portion of its aesthetic appeal. It certainly is the most prominent part of the nose. Made up of two pieces of cartilage called the lower lateral cartilages, they mirror each other on both sides of your nostrils to create the nasal tip. This area determines how long your nose appears in comparison to your other features. When patients come to me concerned about the length of their nose, I have them do an exercise to assess the "tip-defining point." I tell them to stand in front of a mirror with a bright light trained on their nose; the area reflecting the most light is considered the tip-defining point.

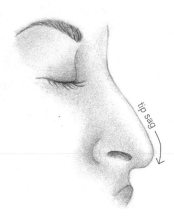

PROFILE OF AN AGING NOSE

The tip structures have separated from the rest of the nose and the tip has drooped. A byproduct of the tip drop is an apparent dorsal hump.

If this point appears too long in relation to the rest of their nose, especially the glabella, the aesthetics of your nose will look out of balance. Width comes into play as well—a nasal tip that is too wide can create imbalance on an otherwise attractive face.

The nasal tip is the one part of your nose susceptible to the effects of aging. As the cartilage of the tip and its connections to the septum start to sag due to gravity, the tip drops and can sometimes develop a "hook" at the end—making the nose appear longer. Skin on the nasal tip can also thicken with age and create a bulbous look (a condition called rhinophyma), which surgery can correct. Just remember that the nasal tip—along with the columella and alar rim—is the most complex area of the nose and therefore should be approached with great care when considering surgical options—whether for alteration or rejuvenation purposes.

COLUMELLA

Most people have to go to a mirror to look for their columella when I explain where it is. But don't be fooled by its seemingly inconspicuous location—the columella has a lot to do with the overall aesthetics of your nose. As with all elements of your nose, a "perfect" columella is determined by its relative position to the features around it. Made up of cartilage and skin, the columella is located between your two nostrils and is comprised of the medial crura of the lower lateral cartilage, which maintains the shape of your nostrils.

The angle between your upper lip and columella is important. For a woman it should be between 95 to 105 degrees (slightly more than a right angle, which allows the nose to tip up a little), while for a man it should be at a perfect 90-degree angle so the nose does not tip up. In addition to its relationship to the upper lip, the columella itself should be slightly bowed—not too straight and not too curved. And a hanging columella (when the columella is overly bowed downward so that the sides are easily seen) is not desirable as it can offer a direct view into your nose from the side. Finally, if the angle between the lip and the columella is greater than 110 degrees the tip will be too high, creating a "Miss Piggy" look.

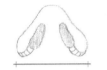

ALAR BASE REDUCTION

A simple surgical technique to narrow a wide alar base by excising a wedge of tissue from each nostril.

ALAR RIM AND ALAR BASE

The alar rim and alar base encompass the bottom area of the nose where your nostrils attach to your cheeks. The alar rim is the upside-down U-shaped edge of your nostril, while the alar base is the width between your two nostrils at your cheek. Again, the desired shape and position of these are determined by the other features of your face as well as your ethnicity. However, within the framework of each ethnic norm (Caucasian, Asian, and black) there are myriad subtle ways to make corrections to the alar rim and alar base without dramatic changes that might end up looking "wrong" on a person. For example, because the underlying cartilage of a wide alar base is stretched, the nostrils have less support and tend to spread out. A good surgeon can reinforce this cartilage, reshaping the nostril without overly altering the alar base and thus staying within ethnic expectations.

Being familiar with these basics of your nasal anatomy will provide you with the ability to communicate clearly with your surgeon and pinpoint the exact areas you feel are in need of correction. Of course, this quick primer is just that—a brief description of the most obvious elements. If your doctor starts using terms that I have not covered, do not panic. Remember, you won't be performing the surgery, he or she will! Again, the most important thing to keep in mind during any consultation for a rhinoplasty is that procedures become more difficult and complex as you move down the nose—and you should now understand why. Thus, any work on the lower third of your nose is going to be more challenging than correcting a small bump on the bone.

GENERAL PROCEDURES AND TECHNIQUES

I have already used the word *artistry* to describe a successful rhinoplasty, and that term should not be taken lightly. A good surgeon not only needs to possess a keen eye for proper balance but, equally important, also has to be able to envision things before they are there. As has been pointed out, the aesthetics of your nose are determined in large part by the relationships among the disparate parts. Therefore, a change in one area can cause a ripple effect in others. A talented doctor should be able to anticipate these subtle shifts and adjust for them. While this type of artistry may prove somewhat difficult to quantify, results are not. Don't be shy about asking to look at "before" and "after" photos so you can determine your surgeon's eye for balance.

Beyond possessing the ability to correctly envision how the nose should look, a good doctor obviously needs the surgical skills to implement that vision—making you more attractive while also protecting the critical functions of your nose. Rhinoplasty is a particularly specialized field with many different techniques used to correct a wide array of problems. Unlike a facelift, where there are three or four top procedures to choose from, working in the nose area requires a large arsenal of surgical skills. The trouble starts when doctors use the same technique—usually the one they learned during their surgical residency—for all rhinoplasties. Just as one key doesn't open up every lock, one surgical solution cannot possibly address all of the subtleties needed in most rhinoplasties. Remember that one out of every seven rhinoplasty patients ends up dissatisfied with the result. Some of these failures are due to particularly difficult operations that—from the outset—were deemed very challenging. But more often than not this high rate of failure is due to surgical inexperience, usually because a "one-size-fits-all" technique was used.

Following is a short description of the three ways rhinoplasties can be performed, all of which offer their own set of pros and cons. The two main differences among them are

caveat emptor

Doctors can use certain photographic tricks to make surgical results look better than they really are—and I am not simply talking about photos that have been noticeably retouched. The shutter speed on a camera can either elongate or shorten a nose depending on where it is set. And bright light in "after" photos can hide problems while low light in "before" photos can magnify them. Here are a few guidelines to follow when looking at a surgeon's "before" and "after" photos:

- Both should be taken from the same distance.

- Both should be taken with the same amount of light; if one picture is yellowish while another is brightly lit, this is a red flag that the photographer is attempting to deceive the viewer.

- Both should be taken with the same facial expression.

- The patient should not be wearing makeup.

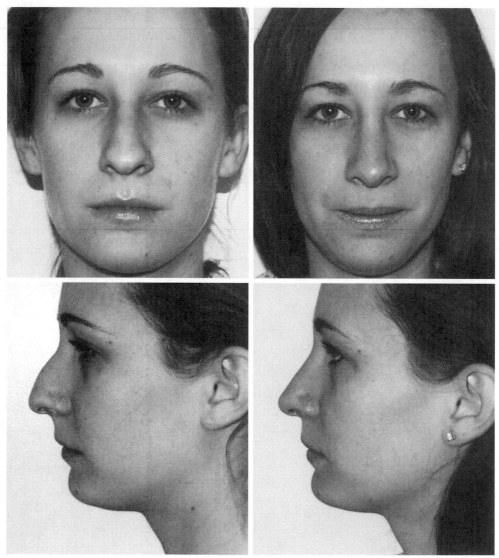

19-YEAR-OLD FEMALE WITH CLOSED RHINOPLASTY

how a surgeon accesses the nose and where the incisions are made. With rhinoplasties, the location of the incision does not just relate to the eventual scar. Rather, the location of the incision also dictates which part of the nose can (and cannot) be worked on during the procedure.

CLOSED RHINOPLASTY

As the name implies, this procedure is performed with minimal invasiveness. Incisions are made inside the nose, a nasal speculum (a tool that spreads the nostril wide open) is inserted, and corrective surgery is performed while the skin is still on the nose. The upside to a closed rhinoplasty is that the swelling is relatively minimal and you will see the final results quickly, in three to six months. The main downside to this type of surgery is that it is not appropriate for a lot of problems, including any issues relating to the tip of the nose. Since the incision is made inside the nose, it is difficult—if not impossible—for the surgeon to go backward toward the tip to make any corrections. Another potential negative to closed rhinoplasty is that it does not allow a surgeon to really see what is happening in the problem area. A good surgeon can make an educated guess as to the exact shape of the deformity, but there is no guarantee that this educated guess will turn out to be right. In a closed rhinoplasty there is no way of confirming what is unseen, so the surgeon must correct the problem a bit "blind." For routine problems of the upper two-thirds of the nose a closed rhinoplasty is as good as the other two techniques. However, for more difficult problems the open technique offers benefits the closed rhino cannot.

OPEN TIP RHINOPLASTY

This is the most precise procedure, allowing the surgeon to treat the entire nose at the same time as well as to see exactly what is happening under the skin. Incisions are made across the columella and then inside the nose at each nasal rim.

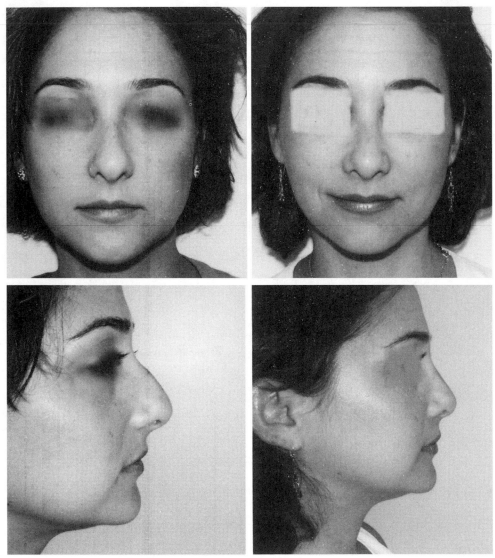

36-YEAR-OLD FEMALE WITH OPEN TIP RHINOPLASTY

Once these incisions have been made the skin is pulled back so that the doctor has surgical access to the entire nose. Having this unobstructed view allows surgeons to better assess what needs to be done and to proceed accordingly. Almost all secondary rhinoplasties are done as open tip rhinoplasties because it offers unfettered access to the problem areas. While the various upsides to this procedure are obvious, the main downside to an open tip rhinoplasty is the swelling that occurs at the tip. Residual swelling can last up to 18 months, making it a serious consideration when weighing your rhinoplasty options. Another downside is the potential for a visible scar across the columella. In an effort to camouflage this, good surgeons will make a stair-step or V-shaped incision on the columella to break up the possible shadow of a straight line. Overall, aside from the few potential problems, this procedure is the best way to maximize results and increase your surgeon's chance of getting your rhinoplasty right the first time.

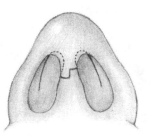

NOSTRILS

Worm's-eye view, with a stair-step columella incision used in an open tip rhinoplasty.

TIP DELIVERY RHINOPLASTY

This is a hybrid procedure designed to combine the benefits of an open tip rhinoplasty with a more closed tip technique. I think it falls short in most cases because there really is no better way to work on a nose than to pull back the skin. But for people who need work

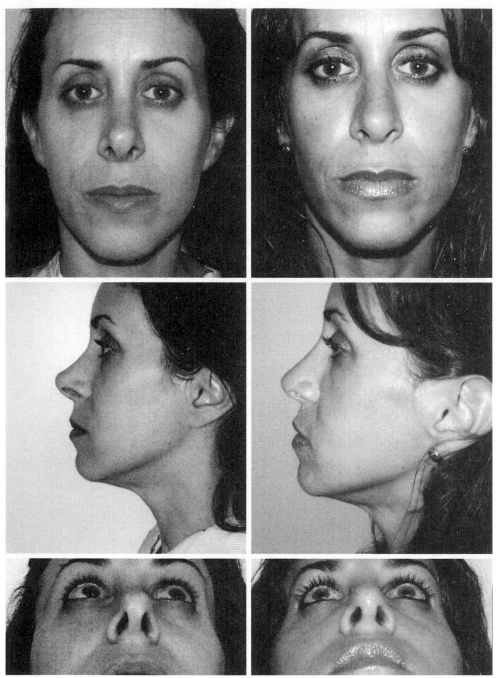

37-YEAR-OLD FEMALE WITH OPEN TIP SECONDARY RHINOPLASTY

Previous rhinoplasty was performed more than 20 years before this procedure.
Midvault was widened with spreader grafts. Tip was lowered and softened.

ankfully, by using computer imaging, I can now illustrate how changing the shape

chin will alter the aesthetics of their nose. Chin implants are a very effective way

ect this type of imbalance. (Chin surgeries are discussed in detail in chapter 6.)

benefit of doing chin surgery combined with a rhinoplasty is that the degree

al change to the shape of the nose will be reduced. And since rhinoplasties are

hat tricky—especially in the tip area—any option that lessens the amount of

lone on the nose while still creating a well-proportioned face is a good thing.

TO EXPECT AFTER A RHINOPLASTY

he procedure, your surgeon will often place a splint on top of the nose to provide

ry support and protection for the traumatized area. It is usual for the splint to

in place for about a week. Some procedures may require a soft, spongelike mate-

be placed in the nasal passages to stop postsurgical bleeding or to add support to

ernal work that was performed. The bleeding should stop within 72 hours, after

the material can be removed.

should expect swelling around the eyes and cheeks. Cold compresses can be used

with the swelling for the first 24 hours postsurgery (along with other medicines

ed in chapter 13). Most important, patients should avoid all nasal traumas for at

x weeks following the surgery—and that includes blowing your nose!

DOES RHINOPLASTY COST?

rhinoplasty is purely cosmetic, then you will probably have to pay for the pro-

yourself as most health insurance covers only those rhinoplasties necessary to

airway issues like a deviated septum. Believe me when I say that you do not

ask your doctor to somehow "fudge" what the true purpose of the procedure is.

performed on the tip and cannot afford a long downtime—celebr

is a decent second choice. A surgeon, by cutting along the top an

lower lateral cartilages, dislodges the cartilage, pulls it out of th

attached to the columella at the alar rim, alters its shape by trim

and then drops it back into its previous position. While the swe

(3 to 12 months), the main problem with this procedure is that

correctly reshape the cartilage because it is not in its natural pos

tion is being done. There are a few circumstances where the tip d

work very well—for example, if the lower lateral cartilages of ea

and there is just a little cartilage to be trimmed and reshaped.

problems I consider it a distant second to the preferred open tip

Rhinoplasty Surgery Type	Swelling	Scar Visibility	Upper ⅔ Nasal Correction
closed	3–6 months	none	++
open tip	6–18 months	possible	+++
tip delivery	3–12 months	none	++

THE CHIN

I have had many patients arrive at their initial consultation compl

too big when the real problem is simply their chin is too weak. Vi

are done to alter the way you look and can be very successful in c

face. Some people are just born with small chins, which can have

making other features seem out of proportion. For example, a ch

prominence can make your nose appear larger than it really is (wh

reading about the chin in a chapter devoted to rhinoplasties).

First, that would be unethical, and I doubt you would feel comfortable trusting your health to a doctor willing to behave in such a way. Second, if the insurance company eventually concludes that the rhinoplasty was cosmetic, then you will be responsible for reimbursing them for any costs they incurred.

The typical cost of a rhinoplasty—including the facility, anesthesia, and surgeon fees—is between $4,000 and $12,000. The price range is wide because it depends on the type of procedure performed, the region of the country, and the experience of the surgeon. Always get a quote that includes all your costs prior to your surgery so there are no hidden surprises. Chin implants—including all fees—usually cost between $2,500 and $5,000.

NOSE AESTHETICS SELF-ASSESSMENT

Is your nose straight? Look directly into a mirror, with light equally distributed on both sides of the nose. Take a ruler or other straightedge and place it against your forehead, in between both eyebrows, then line up the straightedge with the space between your two front teeth. The ruler should split the nose into two equal halves. If you notice a fullness to one side or the other, then your nose is not straight. This can be caused by tip distortion, a deviated septum, upper lateral cartilage collapse, or bony deformities.

Is your profile straight? Take a picture of yourself from the side and enlarge it to a size that is readily examined. Take the same straightedge and place it on the profile of your nose. Does the profile follow the straightedge, or do you see a bump or depression? A nasal bump can be the result of too much bone or cartilage; a depression is likely a result of trauma to this area. If you hold the ruler at the glabella and then pivot it at the nasal tip in both directions, do any of these positions create a more pleasing profile than what you already have?

Is your nose too short or too long? Look directly into a mirror, with light equally distributed on both sides of your nose. There should be a point on the tip of your nose where the light reflection is most visible—this defines the tip of your nose. Your nose can be shortened by lifting the tip up or lengthened by pulling the tip down. The second way to assess the length of your nose is by examining the glabella—that area between your eyes where the nose dips. Some people do not have a well-defined glabella, which makes the nose appear longer.

Is your nose too wide? Or not wide enough? A rule of thumb is that a nose should be narrower between the eyes and widen as it moves down your face toward the tip. Your nostrils, at their widest point, should not be positioned past the inner corner of your eye. A wide nose usually lacks definition and can make your face appear too narrow. Conversely, if your nose does not get wider at the tip it can make your face look fuller than it really is.

Chapter 9

MOUTH AND TEETH

"I've never seen a smiling face that was not beautiful."

—Anonymous

While the eyes are usually the focal point of a face, your mouth and teeth can draw a lot of attention, too. More often than not, if you have healthy teeth and a nicely shaped mouth these features are essentially neutral, neither adding nor subtracting much from your look. Unfortunately, the flip side of this equation is that unsightly problems with your teeth and mouth can seriously diminish the impact of an otherwise beautiful or handsome face. Therefore, it is important to do what you can to keep them both in the best shape possible. Nothing pains me more than to perform a successful facial surgery only to realize that my patient is not planning to correct problems with his or her teeth and mouth. Even the most beautiful, natural-looking facelift will lose some of its "wow factor" without an equally dazzling smile. Thankfully, it is quite common for plastic surgeons and cosmetic dentists to work in concert with each other, very often enhancing the other's work.

This chapter will discuss how aging affects the mouth and teeth and which rejuvenating measures are available to help you reverse those effects. In addition, it will cover the myriad ways in which you can maintain the health of your teeth as well as options for cosmetically enhancing your teeth and mouth. Remember that your smile is an integral part of who you are and is fundamental to how you express yourself. So you should take the time to understand how best to achieve the most perfect smile possible, whether it is by altering your existing features or by rejuvenating those that have diminished over time.

Because a lot of the procedures and treatments covered in this chapter go beyond the scope of plastic surgery, I have consulted with leading dentists who have provided me with accurate, up-to-date information. However, I would advise you to consult with a dentist (or an orthodontist, a periodontist, or an oral surgeon, as necessary) to fully understand the available options related to your particular concerns.

THE IDEAL MOUTH

Before delving into all that can go wrong, it would be helpful to start with a brief description of the necessary elements of an attractive mouth area. As with all things related to plastic surgery, the whole is more than just the sum of its parts. Thus, it is not always enough to have plump red lips and white, straight teeth. Equally important is the relationship between your mouth, lips, and teeth—their relative positioning to each other.

When your mouth is open in a neutral position (neither smiling nor frowning) the vertical height ratio of your lips should be 40 percent upper to 60 percent lower. The corners of your lips should be turned up, with an imaginary line between the two passing through the middle of your upper lip. As you examine the upper lip in this position, 2 to 3 mm of your teeth should be visible from below your upper lip. If any of these elements is not as it should be—for example, your teeth are too long or your lips are too small—the whole mouth can look out of balance and unattractive.

THE EFFECTS OF AGING

As you age, your lips, teeth, and jawbone change. To what degree depends, in large part, on your genetics and lifestyle. The good news is that there are many procedures designed to reverse these changes. Just remember that due to the all-important relative relationship between each element, any one problem can create others. This domino effect can make the task of rejuvenating the mouth area more difficult than one would imagine. However, with the right doctor and dentist, these challenges can most certainly be met.

LIPS

As you age, the white part of your upper lip lengthens in the same way the rest of your skin sags due to gravity and loss of elasticity. This change in shape and position affects the subtle proportions of your face, especially if your upper lip droops enough and begins to conceal your teeth (remember the ideal of showing 2 to 3 mm of teeth). And the more elongated your upper lip becomes, the more your lower lip will appear relatively larger. This can disrupt that optimum 40:60 ratio between the two.

At the same time that the upper lip is getting longer from the nostril sill to the edge of your lip, the red part of your lip is getting thinner. This thinning occurs because the red part of your lip is constantly pulled both horizontally and vertically, which causes atrophy over time. This thinning further disrupts the overall proportions of the mouth area, with the contrast between red and white lip making the change even more obvious.

As the white part of the upper lip lengthens, it puts more force on the lower lip. This can push the lower lip out, creating a pouty look. While that may not sound too bad, once the lower lip starts to move outward, shadows and wrinkles can appear below it.

Another possible effect of aging is that the corners of your lips can start to turn down due to the pull of gravity and the lengthening of the muscles in that area. This can give you a perpetually frowning appearance as well as contribute to the marionette lines on your lower face.

Finally, aging, along with smoking and sun exposure, can cause vertical lines to appear on both the upper and the lower lip. Not only do these make you look older, but they also make it nearly impossible to keep lipstick from bleeding into the skin above the lip. This means that using lipstick to conceal the loss of volume from your upper lip only draws more attention to the problem area.

TEETH

Years of coffee drinking and smoking wreak havoc on your pearly whites—making them yellow or, in extreme cases, brown. Misaligned or crowded teeth can create problems as you age. Beyond the aesthetics, teeth that are in the wrong position are more prone to eventual decay, and they can exacerbate any problems stemming from normal wear and tear. Tooth decay, which can lead to cavities or total loss of the tooth, is usually due to a lack of comprehensive dental hygiene over the years.

Normal wear and tear can result in unattractive chips and cracks. It can also shorten your front teeth, heightening the effect of a lengthening upper lip. The two combined usually conspire to conceal any front teeth during repose. While this type of atrophy is usually due to aging, it can be accelerated by chronic teeth grinding and chemical erosion from gastric reflux disease, excessive consumption of citrus fruits, or bulimia.

Tooth loss can occur due to a variety of reasons—decay, overcrowding, gum disease—most of which can be avoided with good dental hygiene and care. An ounce of prevention really is worth a pound of cure when it comes to your teeth!

BONE

If you have lost teeth throughout the years, as you age you may be more prone to bone loss in your upper and lower jaw. This happens because without the stress from chewing, the bone will atrophy. If bone loss does occur in the jaw, the distance between your nose and chin will get shorter, highlighting the lengthening of your upper lip and pushing out your lower lip and those shadows and wrinkles that come with it.

The temperomandibular joint (TMJ) controls the opening and closing of your jaw. As teeth are lost and the bone stock of the upper and lower jaw recedes, the jaw rotates out and the lower jaw elevates. This causes the bottom portion of your chin to project forward, giving you a "Wicked Witch of the West" look.

All of this may sound a bit bleak, but remember that both genetics and lifestyle determine how aging will affect your lips, mouth, and teeth. Obviously, there is nothing you can do about a genetic predisposition to your jaw rotating out or your upper lip lengthening. Fortunately there are medical procedures available to correct these problems. You can implement a few healthy habits that will help slow the effects of aging as well.

PREVENTATIVE MEASURES

In order to protect the delicate skin and soft tissue of the lip area you need only use a bit of common sense. Smoking, sunbathing, and an unhealthy diet are particularly detrimental to this area, providing yet another reason to stop smoking, avoid excessive sun, and eat a nutritionally balanced diet. The good news is that no matter when you adopt a healthier lifestyle you will reap the rewards, so it is never too late to implement the right habits. In addition, comprehensive skin and lip care can also slow the effects of aging in this area (see chapter 2).

It cannot be overstated how important good dental hygiene is to maintaining a youthful appearance. Beyond the attractiveness of a pearly white smile, healthy teeth help keep everything in place—your lips, jawbone, and chin—as you get older. Thus, if your teeth start to decay or you begin to lose teeth, your lower face will change shape—and it usually does not change for the better! Even if your tooth decay does not reach the point of causing tooth loss, it is still something to be avoided. The weakened enamel of a decaying tooth allows food stains to be more easily absorbed into cracks, causing unattractive discolorations.

Today's marketplace offers many effective products designed to make it easy to take good care of your teeth and gums. These include both home remedies as well as treatments administered by your dentist. Of course, an annual visit to your dentist should be part of any strategy to maintain good dental health.

The American Dental Association advises brushing your teeth twice a day with a soft-bristled toothbrush (medium and hard can be too damaging). It also suggests that you change your toothbrush every six weeks to ensure its effectiveness. As for flossing, the ADA recommends you do it once a day to keep your gums healthy. Gum disease can lead to serious tooth loss, so flossing is essential, even if it is a bit of a grind. My dentist suggested that I do it while watching TV so it feels less time-consuming—and she was right!

There are a few motorized toothbrushes currently on the market that are worth mentioning. The Sonicare Elite uses ultrasound waves to dislodge debris in hard-to-get places around your teeth. The reviews have been good, but some users find it a bit ticklish inside their mouths. The Rota-dent, which has tiny microfibers that rotate at a very high speed, is also designed to clean those hard-to-reach interdental spaces. Keep in mind that motorized toothbrushes should not be viewed as alternatives to flossing since they are unable to clean debris and reduce bacteria below the gum line like flossing does. If motorized toothbrushes are not for you, a good $3 toothbrush and a roll of dental floss is all that is needed.

In addition to daily brushing and flossing, an antibacterial mouthwash can help keep your teeth and gums healthy. Gum disease is caused by bacteria trapped in the gums between your teeth. The resulting infection, gingivitis, can result in inflammation and a receding gum line. Not only is this unattractive, but if the infection is allowed to progress to periodontitis, teeth located near the infected gum can die. By rinsing with an antibacterial mouthwash you increase your chance of loosening debris and killing the bacteria that cause gingivitis. Listerine is still the best over-the-counter choice because it does not contain any sugar (a prime source of acids that promote tooth decay) and it has the highest alcohol content on the market. If you think you already have gingivitis you should see your dentist. Peridex, a prescription mouth rinse, is stronger than Listerine and is best used in this situation. Unfortunately, Peridex can stain your teeth a yellowish brown. Of course, teeth that are slightly yellow are better than no teeth at all—a risk of unchecked gingivitis—so do not let a possible slight discoloration be a deterrent to taking care of your gingivitis. Finally, rinses should not be overused or they can cause dry mouth, which can lead to even more tooth decay!

The final element to your daily brushing, flossing, and rinsing regimen is fluoride. One of Earth's most abundant elements, fluoride protects teeth against the effects of acid and bacteria and helps reverse some initial decay. Luckily, fluoride is present in the majority of U.S. water supplies, so most of us are exposed to its benefits without even trying. But it doesn't hurt to use a fluoride-enhanced toothpaste or rinse if you are looking to boost your protection against tooth decay. And if you are living in an area that does not have fluoride in the water you can speak to your dentist about oral supplements.

caveat emptor — Children under the age of six should not use fluoride-enriched toothpastes or rinses. Fluorosis, which can stain teeth a yellow-brown, is caused when young children have too much fluoride in their diet. Since kids might very well swallow a rinse or toothpaste, it is best to avoid fluoride-enriched products until they are seven years old.

There is one final preventative measure that needs mentioning. Bruxism, which is the habitual grinding of teeth while you sleep, must be addressed or it may result in shortened, cracked, or broken teeth. While it is difficult to stop grinding your teeth, it is possible to protect those teeth from damage. The most effective way to do this is with a custom-made nightguard appliance. Your dentist can fit you with one that allows for a normal bite between your upper and lower jaws while avoiding any gum irritation. A well-fitted guard not only protects your teeth but also relaxes the chewing muscles, reducing the lactic acid buildup that normally accompanies teeth-grinding. Patients report fewer headaches (migraines included) and less muscle spasm as a result of this reduction in lactic acid buildup. A nightguard appliance also helps align your jaw properly while you sleep, keeping your temperomandibular joint healthy. Just be mindful of the fact that wearing an *ill-fitted* mouth guard can throw off your bite, resulting in an irritation to the TMJ joint and possibly doing more damage than the bruxism itself! Therefore, most dentists strongly advise avoiding over-the-counter guards as they usually do not fit properly.

FIXING THE PROBLEMS

Whether your problems are due to the effects of aging or bad habits or are simply features you have always been unhappy with, there are a lot of options available—running the gamut from over-the-counter solutions to surgical procedures—that can make your teeth, lips, and mouth look more attractive. If you are considering some of the more complicated procedures involving your teeth and the soft tissue of your face, you should consult both a plastic surgeon and a cosmetic dentist.

ELONGATED UPPER LIP

A lip lift is really the only effective way to reverse a sagging upper lip. Both the red and the white part of the upper lip are lifted by making an incision at the base of the nostrils, resecting some skin and soft tissue below the incision, and then reattaching the skin by lifting it to the base of the nostril. This procedure is relatively straightforward and usually heals without a hitch. If done properly there should be no visible scar.

TURNED-DOWN LIP CORNERS

Botox injections can be used to correct turned-down lips by weakening the muscles responsible for pulling down the corners. Just remember that, as is the case with most Botox applications, less is more. The goal is to soften the downturn, not make it impossible for you to frown if you want to. If your doctor uses too strong a dose, the paralyzed muscles won't allow you to communicate nonverbal displeasure.

A surgical procedure can also be done to lift the corners of the mouth. An incision is made on the edge of the red of your lip at each corner. A small triangle of skin is excised and then the skin is sutured, thereby lifting the corners of your mouth. The only downside to this procedure is the possibility of a visible scar because there is no place to conceal it. But if stitched properly more than likely the scar will be imperceptible.

GUMMY SMILE

If too much gum shows when you smile, a periodontist can lift the height of your gums. This is done by removing a small amount of gum tissue at the top of the tooth. By exposing more of the tooth, your smile becomes better proportioned and your teeth appear to be the correct length. If your teeth end up looking too long after the gum has been elevated your dentist can shorten the teeth as well.

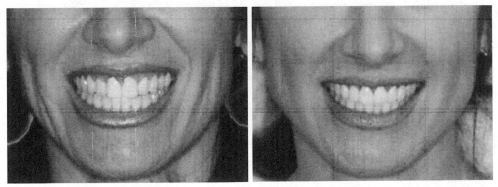

CORRECTION OF A GUMMY SMILE

The exposed gum above the teeth is improved by elevating the gums and adding new veneers with a slightly shorter tooth length. (Photos courtesy of Dr. Timothy Chase.)

Considerably more involved than a gum lift, a bone manipulation procedure surgically shortens the height of the upper jawbone. The surgeon makes a horizontal cut into the bone above the tooth, removes a portion of the bone equal to the desired amount of elevation, and then reattaches the two pieces of bone together. There is more risk to this procedure—risk that most practitioners consider unnecessary since the gum lift can usually achieve the same results.

WRINKLED LIPS

Injected in small amounts, Botox can be effective in weakening the muscles that cause these pesky smokers' lines. However, be mindful of the fact that paralyzing the muscles that cause the wrinkles may also make your mouth feel overly stiff and frozen—so the dose has to be small.

Fillers can also be used to get rid of lip wrinkles, by injecting either small amounts directly into the wrinkle or larger amounts into the lip, plumping it up so the wrinkles disappear. Sometimes a doctor will inject a thin bead of filler at the junction between the red and white skin of the lip. This helps push out the wrinkles as well as give more volume to the upper lip. Just make sure your doctor doesn't overdo it or you may end up looking like Daffy Duck.

Some skin care products may offer relief for wrinkled lips. Antioxidants, retinoic acid treatments, and alpha hydroxy acid treatments are all somewhat effective in lessening the appearance of these fine lines. Please refer to chapter 3 for more on effective skin care products for the lips.

Some lipsticks are formulated to increase blood flow to your lips, temporarily making them fuller and as a result getting rid of the wrinkles, at least for a while. These lipsticks might not offer a long-term solution, but they can't hurt. And they do prevent your lipstick from bleeding into the skin of your upper lip.

DIMINISHING UPPER LIP

Fillers can be used to increase the volume of your lips. They can be injected throughout the lip or as a thin bead at the junction between the red and white border skin of the lip. Again, just make sure the doctor does not overdo it as this can push your lip out, making it appear almost bill-like. Keep in mind that fillers are not permanent, so the procedure will have to be repeated as long as you want a more voluminous look. Fillers should not be used to add more volume on an older person who is dealing with a lengthening upper lip, as it will just exacerbate the appearance of the elongation. This is a point that needs repeating because older patients who have had successful results with fillers on other parts of their face understandably would like the same results on their lips. I must remind them that anything that elongates the lip (even if it gets rid of fine lines) will only make them look older.

There are also surgical procedures that offer a more permanent way to add volume to your lips. You can choose to use your own tissue (fat, dermis, or tendon) to add volume or you can opt to have a synthetic lip plumper implanted.

Fat. This is probably the simplest of the three tissue options and is gaining in popularity because it is soft and natural looking. Your fat, extracted by a needle through a pinhole anywhere on your body, is processed and then injected into your lips. The procedure is basically risk free and only requires a local anesthesia. The one downside to using fat is that it does not always last. If it does, however, most patients are extremely satisfied with the results. The Viafill System is a newer technique designed to provide longer-lasting results.

Dermis. This deep layer of the skin is soft, durable, and malleable. Surgeons will shape it into a sausage-like implant and then thread it through your lip. The blood supply from the lip will grow into the dermis, making the implant last a very long time. While longevity is a plus, there are a number of downsides to using dermis for this purpose. First, the donor site from which the skin is harvested will usually result in a scar. Second, the sausage-like graft can end up looking and feeling unnatural. Finally, on occasion patients can develop uncomfortable and unsightly cysts within the graft, requiring additional surgery to fix the problem. I no longer perform dermis lip implants because of this potential complication.

Tendon. This is being hailed as a new procedure with long-lasting and natural results. The procedure is similar to the dermis implant. Tendons from the wrist are harvested and then threaded into the lip. The first drawback of using tendons for this implant is that you are left with a scar on your wrist where it was harvested. Second, although the doctor uses a non-essential tendon, patients are not thrilled with giving up a wrist tendon for a cosmetic procedure, especially when there are other viable options. Finally, the tendon implant can end up feeling somewhat cordlike, which can make kissing an adventure!

Synthetic Lip Implants. Gore-Tex and cadaveric dermis implants have continued to be problematic. They can look unnatural, are prone to infection, and can sometimes extrude to the point of requiring removal. A newer synthetic implant, which is an inflatable balloon, may look more natural (read: less hard) but has not been around long enough to fully understand the pros and cons of the procedure. Thus, my advice is to avoid synthetic implants altogether and stick with either temporary fillers or fat injections if you are looking to increase the volume of your upper lip.

While most patients undergoing lip surgery are looking to repair the effects of aging, some patients are interested in simply altering the lips with which they were born. More often than not this involves a lip reduction, and the target area is usually the lower lip. A lip reduction is a relatively easy fix that can be performed with local anesthesia. Horizontal cuts are made inside the lip, excess skin and tissue are removed, and then the incisions are closed, leaving little to no scars inside the mouth.

DISCOLORED TEETH

Smoking, drinking, and eating will all result in a slow staining of your pearly whites. A once-beautiful smile can be severely diminished with brown or yellow stains on the teeth. The basic treatment for these problems is chemical bleaching. How effective the results are will be determined by the degree of staining as well as the strength of the bleach used. There are many options for whitening discolored teeth, either at home or in the dentist's office. Some widely available at-home tooth whiteners include:

Whitening Toothpastes. Typically costing under $10 per tube, whitening toothpastes can help correct slightly discolored teeth. My informal survey among dentists found that the three best bests are Pearl Drops Whitening Toothpaste, Arm & Hammer Advance White Baking Soda and Peroxide Toothpaste, and Aquafresh whitening toothpaste. Apparently, the other more costly products that are being heavily promoted are not worth your hard-earned dollars. Keep in mind that whitening toothpastes are better used as follow-up maintenance after undergoing a stronger whitening procedure such as those described below.

Whitening Strips. Offering low concentrations of carbamide peroxide (a whitener), these cellophane strips affix to your teeth for daily treatments. Because they are sold over the counter, the concentration level is designed to prevent you from doing damage to your lips and gums. Unfortunately, this low concentration also means that you will not see much in the way of teeth whitening. Anecdotal evidence suggests that they are not worth the cost, effort, and discomfort of applying them for a half hour every day.

Gel-filled Trays. These trays, which you can purchase over the counter for $30 to $50, are filled with a low dose of carbamide peroxide that you keep on your teeth for 30 minutes or so. A gel tray is not a bad way to follow up an in-office whitening treatment, but because of the low concentration of carbamide peroxide the overall whitening results will be minimal if used on its own.

For those patients truly motivated to correct seriously discolored teeth, dentist's office whitening procedures can offer rather startling results—at a premium price, of course.

Carbamide Peroxide 35 Percent Gel. Clinical studies have shown this treatment to whiten teeth by six shades of color and to last for up to five years. To further enhance the treatment, your dentist may fit you with a custom dental tray so you can apply carbamide peroxide while you sleep. These custom gel trays, about one-third the strength of an in-office whitening, are worn one or two times a day for two weeks following the in-office treatment. Studies suggest that custom trays, when combined with office procedures, yield better results than all other treatments. The only problem with custom trays is that patients may not use them as regularly as prescribed, diminishing the overall results.

Carbamide Peroxide Gel with a Special Light. This is the same treatment as above, but the chemical reaction of the whitening agent is enhanced by a special light (marketed under the names Zoom or Bright Smile) applied during the procedure. Some studies have shown that this special light does not add much to the whitening effect of the carbamide peroxide. Therefore, instead of paying extra for the light application, it is probably a better idea to follow up the carbamide peroxide treatment with the doctor-prescribed home gel treatments described above.

Laser Tooth Lightening. Most dentists I spoke with think this procedure offers more hype than results and that it is overpriced.

MISALIGNED OR CROWDED TEETH

Orthodontia, the practice of using braces to straighten teeth, is no longer just for kids. If you missed the opportunity for braces while growing up, it is not too late! Orthodontia is important for both aesthetic reasons and to protect your teeth from accelerated tooth decay or loss. There are two newer options that offer adults a less embarrassing way to endure the one to two years required for treatment.

Inside Braces. These are attached to the back of your teeth and are not visible. The one complaint dentists hear is that they can be a bit uncomfortable.

Invisalign. These are clear plastic dental trays that are custom-designed for your teeth. A patient wears the tray constantly and every two weeks the tray is replaced by one that is a slightly different size. Over the course of six months to a year these trays gently push your teeth into alignment.

TOOTH DECAY

Various fillings can be used to deal with tooth decay. Prior to filling a cavity, a dentist must use a drill to carve out all of the tooth decay. If the decay has traveled to the soft root of the tooth, a root canal must be done prior to filling the area.

Amalgam. These fillings are what most people over 40 are accustomed to. They are silver in color and can be quite obvious if a person has a mouth full of them. While amalgam fillings are extremely durable and can be done in one visit, they have mercury in them. Even though all studies have shown that amalgam is not dangerous, with newer alternatives on the market the use of amalgam is in decline.

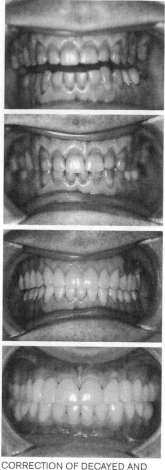

CORRECTION OF DECAYED AND
DAMAGED TEETH WITH VENEERS
(Photos courtesy of Dr. Steven Roth.)

Gold Fillings. While safe and durable, gold is expensive and requires more than one office visit for placement. They can also be a bit too shiny, which might be considered unattractive by some patients.

Acrylic Resins. These fillings are popular because they are safe and cost effective and can be done in one office visit. The downside to acrylic resin fillings is that they will eventually wear down, especially in high-stress areas.

CHIPPED OR CRACKED TEETH

Chipped or cracked teeth can be repaired with porcelain veneers and crowns. A veneer is a facade of porcelain that is glued across the entire front and side borders of your teeth, with your own teeth acting as the anchor. Crowns, which are applied to the sides and the bite area of your teeth, are usually used on your grinding molars. Porcelain is extremely strong and durable with a nice translucent quality to it, making these veneers and crowns the top choice of many dentists. The downsides of using porcelain are that it can crack or chip, is very expensive, and requires more than one office visit to do the work. Acrylic resins can also be used to repair small cracks and chips (a process called "bonding"), but resin is less translucent than porcelain, so these fixes can sometimes look fake or off-color.

LOSS OF TEETH

Dentures, bridges, and osteointegrated implants are available options to correct the loss of teeth.

Dentures are false teeth that are attached to a substrate, which is glued to your gums. The drawbacks to dentures are numerous: they can fall out at embarrassing times, they must removed before sleeping, they can make speaking and chewing difficult, they can cause soreness and irritation to the gums, and they can create bad breath.

A bridge is a denture or dentures attached to healthy teeth on either side of the gap. The drawbacks of bridges are the same as those of dentures, although probably to a slightly lesser degree since they are anchored to other teeth.

Osteointegrated implants offer a more permanent alternative to dentures and bridges. An anchor is drilled into the bone, the bone eventually grows over the anchor, and then a false tooth is attached to the anchor by a post. Because the false tooth is permanently fixed in position, the tooth does not move or fall out. And since it is attached at the gum line, the false tooth looks extremely natural. An important long-term benefit to these implants is that the stress placed on the jawbone by chewing ensures a strong jawbone that will not atrophy, which can be a problem as you age. Osteointegrated implants are considerably more expensive than dentures or bridges. And if done improperly, anchor failure or infection can be problems. But these issues seem to be the very small exception rather than the rule.

DENTISTRY OR PLASTIC SURGERY?

In order to get help from the appropriate professional you will need to correctly assess the problems in your mouth area. If your mouth is closed and you are unhappy with the shape or size of your lips or you notice excessive wrinkling in the area, then you should see a plastic surgeon. If your mouth is open and you are displeased by the shape, color,

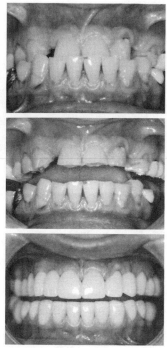

TOTAL MOUTH RECONSTRUCTION
WITH VENEERS AND
OSTEOINTEGRATED IMPLANTS

(Photo courtesy of Dr. Kenneth
Fishman.)

or position of your teeth, then you should seek out a great dentist. And remember that it is not uncommon for dentists and plastic surgeons to work together if your particular situation demands it.

HOW MUCH DOES IT COST?

Although most chapters in this book end with a brief outline of the cost of procedures that have been discussed, this chapter is too broad to do so. But I will note that, more so than in any other area covered in this book, an ounce of prevention is most worth a pound of cure. Good dental hygiene is a lot cheaper than fixing any problems that stem from bad dental hygiene. So brush and floss daily, visit your dentist once a year, and you will save your teeth as well as a lot of money.

Internet Resources: Dentistry

www.ada.org/public/index.asp

Chapter 10

EARS

"Everything has beauty, but not everyone sees it."

—Confucius

For most of us, a beautiful ear is one that is unobtrusive. If you notice it, then it must be too big or prominent. Although the problem of prominent ears may be most troubling for children, there are certainly many adults concerned about the shape and size of their ears. In contrast to a prominent ear caused by genetics, aging brings about few changes to the aesthetics of the ears, with the exception of hanging or stretched out earlobes. This chapter will discuss the options for correction of prominent ears, as well as the treatment of earlobes and their ornaments.

PROTRUDING EARS

We all know that kids can be mean. And ears that stick out tend to be easy targets for merciless teasing and cruel nicknames. This condition is especially difficult for boys because, unlike girls, they cannot hide their ears behind long hair. Growing up with protruding ears does not cause any medical problems; the condition's harmful effects are measured in psychological terms, which can be just as damaging to a young person's development as a physical ailment.

Thankfully, fixing ears that protrude is a relatively minor procedure that can be performed in a doctor's office with local anesthesia. And if the operation is done at the right time the child can avoid any long-term emotional scarring. In my opinion, there are very few downsides to an otoplasty, with much more to lose if it is not performed.

TIMING AN OTOPLASTY

The proper timing of a childhood otoplasty depends on three factors. First, the operation should not be performed before the ears have grown close to adult size, at six to eight years of age. If an otoplasty is done before this time the procedure might cause aesthetic problems as the ear continues to grow. Second, it is probably time to think of correcting the problem if the teasing has escalated and the youngster is being particularly brutalized. Finally, the child must be emotionally ready to make the change and be open to the idea of the otoplasty.

As you age, the cartilage in the ear becomes less malleable, making adult procedures slightly different in order to account for this decrease in the bendability. But keep in mind that even the most complicated otoplasty is quite straightforward, presenting little or no risk to the patient.

ANATOMY AND PROCEDURES

There are two possible causes of protruding ears. Either the conchal bowl is too large and is pushing the rest of the ear away from the head, or the usual bend in the outer ear cartilage—the antihelix—is missing and that causes the ear to flop forward. Sometimes protruding ears are due to a combination of both.

If the conchal bowl (the part of the ear that you can stick your finger into that looks like a bowl) is too big, a surgeon will make it smaller by cutting out some of the skin and cartilage through an incision behind the ear. Once that is done the surgeon may find it necessary to stitch the bowl to a spot behind the ear, helping it stay in place closer to the head.

Fixing the antihelix is slightly more complicated in that a surgeon must add a crease to the existing cartilage and do so in a natural-looking way that is durable. The antihelix can be created artificially by tightly stitching along a line behind the ear where the fold should have been. These "pinching" sutures will form a crease and force the outer ear back toward the head. Previously, plastic surgeons would create the fold by cutting right through the cartilage and then stitching it back up at an angle. This is no longer considered a viable option because it can give the cartilage sharp edges, making it appear unnatural (which, of course, the fold is). If a surgeon suggests this procedure you should probably get another opinion.

One of the first otoplasties I ever performed made me feel like a character in a Frank Capra movie. My patient, a 10-year-old boy, had been playing on the street outside his New York apartment with some friends. Just as an older gentleman was passing by, a few of the boys started teasing the youngster about his ears. The man saw how hurtful this teasing was and felt compelled to do something. He found the boy's mother and promised to pay for the procedure to fix her son's ears—a promise he kept. It turns out that the older gentleman had suffered through his own childhood with protruding ears, finally fixing them later in life, and wanted to protect this young boy from the same fate. I tell you the story not only because it is a heartwarming tale of a stranger's kindness, but also because it is a strong indication of how deeply scarring this kind of intense teasing can be.

WHAT TO EXPECT WITH EAR SURGERY

The actual otoplasty is relatively straightforward and pain free. The challenge is in protecting the repaired ear after the surgery. Since the cartilage is under some stress, any force that works against the sutures can cause them to rip, reversing the benefits of the procedure. Remember that the cartilage will be bent and following the surgery will be held together with stitches.

There are two important things to be careful of during the convalescence period. First, damage can be done to the sutures at night from any twisting movement against a pillow. Therefore, the patient should go to bed wearing a headdress for the first two weeks, followed by a sweatband over the ears for the next six weeks. Second, children may continue to tease the patient even after the operation, and in doing so may try to flick the ear forward or bend it in some way. I advise all of my younger patients to wear a sweatband over their ears to protect against this type of unfortunate behavior. It also helps for the parent to send a note to the school so teachers can be on the lookout for bullying.

AM I A CANDIDATE FOR THE PROCEDURE?

Aside from the typical child with severely prominent ears, I often have patients in their twenties who did not have the surgery when they were younger but are now aware of a modest prominence to their ears. They come to me a bit embarrassed, unsure if their ears even merit surgery. The beauty of this procedure is that improvements can be made with minimal discomfort and limited risks, so if there is any chance of benefiting from an otoplasty it is best to schedule a consultation with a plastic surgeon.

EARLOBES AND PIERCING

I occasionally see patients with earlobe problems. Either their lobes have become disfigured or torn from wearing heavy earrings or their lobes are just naturally oversized. Most procedures to fix the earlobe are relatively minor and are done under local anesthesia in a doctor's office. If your earlobe is torn, a surgeon will remove the skin in the tunnel of the opening, stitch the hole together, and then close it over. If you have naturally large earlobes, a surgeon will cut out a small wedge from the lobe and then stitch it up. The only caveat to repairing an earlobe is that it can never be pierced again in the same place because the scar tissue from the repair is not as strong as your own healthy tissue and a new piercing would reopen the tear in the earlobe.

I think it is important to mention that piercing the cartilage of the upper ear is dangerous and should be avoided. This area of the ear has a smaller blood supply than the earlobe, so it is more prone to becoming infected and causing problems down the line. So now when your teenager asks to have this done you can offer a legitimate medical reason for saying no!

caveat emptor

Probably 99.9 percent of all ear piercings are done at the local jewelry store by someone with minimal training. While the procedure is usually safe, the piercing is often done in the wrong place on the earlobe and in the wrong direction. To best showcase earrings—especially studs—the hole should be directed so that the earring faces forward. This way if someone is looking straight at you he would be able to see those gorgeous diamond studs you're wearing. At the same time, the piercing should be done high to low (i.e., the hole in the back of your earlobe should be slightly lower than the opening in the front). By doing so, heavier studs will be "propped up" slightly and not droop as easily.

HOW MUCH DOES IT COST?

The cost of an otoplasty usually runs from $3,000 to $6,000, depending on the patient's geographic location, the experience of the surgeon, and the type of repair to be performed. Procedures to fix torn earlobes can run from $400 to $1,000.

Chapter 11

HAIR

"The hair is the richest ornament of woman."

—Martin Luther

J ust like a beautiful painting, your face is greatly enhanced when it is framed properly. A healthy head of hair that is appropriately styled can complement your features and add polish to your overall look. Thankfully, in today's marketplace there are a number of options and products available to make a great head of hair a reality. Of course, there is also a considerable amount of hype—especially when it comes to the problem of hair loss—so you will need to be a savvy consumer to get the most for your money.

This chapter will provide you with a basic primer on the causes of thinning hair, helping you to understand which remedies are most likely to work. If medicine is not able to reverse your hair loss, I discuss what your best surgical options are. Finally, there is a section on how to make the most of the hair that you do have with tips on styling, color, and cut.

CAUSES OF HAIR LOSS

While the vast majority of baldness and hair loss is genetic (85 percent) the remaining causes are disease (most notably thyroid irregularities), radiation and chemotherapy used on cancer patients, and various forms of bodily stress such as excessive weight loss or pregnancy. The appropriate treatments for each will differ, so it is important to identify what is causing your hair loss to effectively solve the problem. In most instances of disease and stress-related baldness, the follicle is not permanently damaged, so your hair can grow back again after the underlying cause has been remedied. Androgenetic hair loss—that which is determined by your genes—presents more of a challenge because the problematic follicles may be damaged beyond repair, rendering them unable to produce hair again.

Hair loss manifests itself in two distinct ways: patchy and generalized. Localized patches of baldness are usually temporary and easier to treat than generalized hair loss, which, as the term implies, occurs throughout the scalp. But overall hair loss is no longer the bleak condition it was fifty years ago. Great strides have been made in reversing generalized hair loss through a better understanding of the hormonal irregularities that underlie the condition.

Before going any further it might be a good idea to identify the normal cycles of hair loss and growth so you can better understand what is happening when problems occur. At any given time, 10 percent of your hair follicles are dormant and do not produce hair. This is cyclical, with each follicle resting after being active for three years. Standard hair loss is about 100 hairs a day, and regular hair growth is about half an inch per month. You have a lot of hair follicles on your head, so it takes a while for generalized hair loss to become noticeable. In fact, studies have shown that by the time most people recognize they have a problem 50 percent of their hair is already gone!

PATCHY HAIR LOSS

There are four types of localized hair loss—some more common than others. The good news is that all are completely reversible.

Alopecia Areata. This is a condition of patchy bald spots, usually the size of a quarter, that happens in a few different places on the scalp and is caused by an autoimmune irregularity (when the body attacks itself for no apparent reason). Alopecia areata is one of those oddities of the human body that is self-limiting and usually burns itself out. Thus, the best treatment is to do nothing and use your existing hair to conceal the few bald patches.

Traction Alopecia. When hair is pulled too tightly it can damage the follicle and cause hair loss. The only course of treatment is to get rid of the traction. Once that is done, the follicle usually repairs itself and hair starts growing again. Certain hairstyles, such as cornrows or tight braids, are the main culprits of traction alopecia, so they are to be avoided if you want to maintain a healthy head of hair.

Trichotillomania. You probably remember someone telling you to stop playing with your hair when you were growing up. For good reason! Any type of excessive pulling, twisting, or biting of your hair can result in hair loss. Since this is a nervous disorder, only a mental health practitioner can offer proper treatment. Once the compulsive behavior stops, the hair usually grows back.

Tinea Capitis. Sometimes a fungus can attack your scalp and temporarily damage the follicle. Symptoms include an itchy, flaky scalp as well as hair loss. This is not a particularly common problem, but a good dermatologist will be able to diagnose the condition. The best treatment is the use of anti-fungal creams applied directly to the scalp. Once the fungus has been killed the hair grows back. Note that many of the symptoms of tinea capitis are the same as dandruff or eczema. An effective treatment depends on diagnosing the problem correctly, so it really is important to seek a professional opinion if you suspect you may have a fungal infection of the scalp.

GENERALIZED HAIR LOSS

There are two types of generalized hair loss—telogen effluvium and androgenetic alopecia. The first is stress related and the second is genetically determined. Both types

It should be pointed out that since testosterone travels slightly different paths in men and women, the medical treatments used to reverse male-pattern baldness cannot be used to reverse female-pattern baldness. In fact, it is actually dangerous to do so. This type of gender-specific treatment is quite rare in medicine, so it is worth noting, especially in today's world of Internet self-cures.

One last word on treatments: If you do not see it listed here, then it is not worth your hard-earned money! There is still an enormous amount of hype surrounding baldness and its cures. You need to educate yourself to ensure you choose the right treatment—not only to protect your wallet but also to protect your psyche. Losing one's hair can be rife with emotion and the last thing you need is to be preyed upon by unscrupulous marketers hawking false hopes.

MINOXIDIL

This topical lotion or foam—equally appropriate for women and men—comes in two strengths (2 percent and 5 percent) and is rubbed into your scalp twice a day. A doctor will usually start you at 2 percent and then increase it to 5 percent once the regrowth starts to wane after regular use. Minoxidil does reverse hair loss but usually does not bring back all of the follicles, so the results can be mixed. It also takes time—up to two months—to see any noticeable improvement. The interesting thing about minoxidil is that it is still somewhat of a mystery as to why it actually works. Studies have shown that it does not affect DHT (which is the underlying cause of androgenetic alopecia), so the way in which it repairs the follicle is unclear. The main problem with minoxidil is that because it takes time and requires twice-daily applications that can get messy, a lot of people give up on it before they actually see results. A recently introduced foam version was designed, in large part, to make this less of a problem.

PROPECIA

Exclusively for men, this treatment is taken as a daily pill, which blocks your body from turning testosterone into DHT. It can be used in conjunction with minoxidil with usually strong results. Propecia will stop the progression of more follicles closing up, while minoxidil repairs some of those already damaged. As is the case with minoxidil, if you stop using Propecia your baldness will continue to progress. The upside to Propecia is that it does not require twice-daily applications of a messy lotion or foam. The downside is that it can cause impotence or lack of libido, which is not a minor consideration. Under no circumstance should women take Propecia—it has the potential to cause birth defects in male fetuses.

ALDACTONE

Like Propecia, Aldactone is a pill—prescribed only for female-pattern baldness—that blocks the creation of DHT. Studies have shown that women respond extremely well to this treatment, with 88 percent of Aldactone patients experiencing improvement. Aldactone can be taken in conjunction with minoxidil, offering a two-pronged assault on hair loss in the same way Propecia and minoxidil work together to treat male-pattern baldness. The Aldactone slows down the effects of DHT, while the Minoxidil helps bring some follicles back to life. You should be aware that Aldactone can affect blood pressure (it is used as a medication for high blood pressure), so any patient seeking to treat her alopecia with Aldactone should be monitored by a physician.

HAIR TRANSPLANTS

Regarding the latest technology in hair transplantation, I spoke with world-renowned dermatologist Dr. Joel Kassimir, who has worked on thousands of high-profile patients. He told me, "The science behind successful hair transplantation has been figured out, but the real challenge is in understanding the artistry involved in the process." While it may be true that many transplant patients have ended up with an unfortunate cornfield look, the good news is that if done correctly, today's transplants (called "mini plugs" or "micrografts") can appear totally natural.

Hair transplants are performed by harvesting patches of your own skin from areas of your scalp where hair is still growing and regrafting these to your bald areas. The harvesting and regrafting are done in the same session. In the pioneering days of this surgery the grafts were large (with 10 to 15 follicles each) and were often "planted" in rows, creating the aforementioned cornfield look. Today the grafts are much smaller and placed irregularly so there is no obvious pattern (mini plugs have two or three hair follicles, while micrografts have a single follicle). Surgeons can now use different-size grafts with varying numbers of hair follicles to create an even more natural look. Another recent improvement is that transplanted follicles are now placed at angles that mimic nearby follicles, so they no longer appear to have been just pasted onto the scalp. The surgery is labor-intensive—both harvesting the grafts and transplanting them—so a large area usually requires multiple sessions in your doctor's office. Most hair transplants are done by general surgeons or dermatologists, not plastic surgeons.

Dr. Kassimir points out that men should not wait until they have a bald head to look into a hair transplant. Although you can still have transplants at this later stage, his advice is to start earlier, before all of the frontal hair falls out, in order to achieve the best possible result.

The main benefit of a hair transplant, in comparison to other treatments, is that you end up with a natural-looking head of hair that should last without further treatment. Additionally, there is minimal discomfort associated with the procedure. The downsides are that the procedure can be costly and there is a small chance the follicles that have been regrafted may close up as well, since androgenetic alopecia is progressive.

This surgery works just as well for women as it does for men. In fact, because female-pattern baldness is more a problem of thinning hair, transplants on women tend to produce particularly natural results. The pros and cons are the same for women as they are for men—it is a tedious, costly process but one that usually produces the most long-lasting results.

Dr. Kassimir notes that transplants for women can be done in a variety of different ways depending on the needs of the patient. For those with generalized loss of hair, grafting can be performed throughout the scalp or at the hairline as a form of camouflage. And for patients who have had facelifts, brow lifts, or other procedures, grafting at the hairline is particularly helpful in concealing any visible scars.

SCALP REDUCTION

This surgery, which has always been considered rather drastic, is now becoming obsolete since hair transplants are producing such natural results. Basically, a scalp reduction involves swapping the bald scalp at the front of the head with scalp still growing hair at the back of the head. The first problem with this procedure is that the direction of the hair follicles looks unnatural. However, the main problem is the scars—if the hairline were to recede further there would be no way of hiding them. You really should not consider this surgery, and if a doctor suggests it I would advise you to seek medical treatment elsewhere.

ARTIFICIAL HAIR

Finally, though not considered an actual treatment, both men and women with thinning hair can invest in hairpieces or wigs. This may be a good option if your scalp is not responding to medical treatment or you are not interested in or cannot afford a hair transplant. Some companies now offer natural-looking pieces that can withstand an active lifestyle. If you decide to go this route, my advice would be to choose very carefully—there are big differences in the quality of products currently being offered.

Also, it is critical to make certain the color of your hair and the hairpiece match perfectly or it is going to look very phony.

HAIR HEALTH AND DIET CONNECTION

The old adage "you are what you eat" is particularly true when it comes to your hair. Biotin, a B vitamin, is fundamental to maintaining a healthy head of hair. A biotin deficiency can result in very dry hair, hair breakage, and a cracking scalp. Good dietary sources of biotin are egg yolks, liver, cheese, and lobsters. Of course, you can also take biotin supplements—300 micrograms a day is the recommended dosage (pregnant women should take 350 micrograms). If you are eager to provide your dry hair with a real boost, you can increase the micrograms considerably. Since biotin is water soluble, whatever cannot be absorbed will simply flush out of your system. Studies have shown that antacids can block your body's absorption of biotin, so if you have noticed a sudden problem of dryness with your scalp or hair you should monitor your consumption of these.

STYLING

If you are faced with thinning hair there are a few tricks you can employ to give it more volume. A haircut with layers can usually create the illusion of thicker hair, especially if you brush your hair rather than comb it every day. And when blow-drying your hair you should use the cooler setting, which adds loft to thin hair (the hotter the setting the straighter and flatter the hair will become). Many of the new volumizing shampoos and conditioners on the market have been shown to work. If you are fair-skinned, lightening your hair will make any exposed scalp less noticeable. Finally, a curly perm can give the impression of much thicker hair.

PART THREE

Journey to
Beauty

Chapter 12

SELECTING A PLASTIC SURGEON

"Beauty and Folly are generally companions."

—Baltasar Gracian

N ow that you have read through this book you may find yourself eager to set up a consultation appointment with a plastic surgeon. But where do you start? Unless you live in a particularly remote area, the sheer volume of practices vying for your business (and dollars) will probably be overwhelming. This chapter will help you cut through the hype. By using my clearly defined set of criteria as a guide, you should have no problem finding a properly trained, fully accredited plastic surgeon who will be right for you.

EDUCATION AND ACCREDITATION

As is the case in most professions, there is a training hierarchy in plastic surgery. Our field has its top schools, highly rigorous residency programs, and hard-won positions in leading hospitals. This is not to say that a great plastic surgeon cannot come out of a middling program. But students at the best schools usually have an edge in that they are exposed to and influenced by the best teachers in the field.

Studying to be a board-certified plastic surgeon is a grueling and lengthy process. At each stage in their medical training, students either excel or they don't. And programs are designed to ensure that those who move forward are the most committed and talented of their group. The demands of a plastic surgery program are intense, and many students simply cannot keep up. By the time a doctor is finished with his or her training it is not unusual for them to be in their late thirties or early forties.

4 years of college

4 years of medical school

3–5 years of surgical training

2–3 years of plastic surgery training

1–2 years of specialization training within plastic surgery

what it takes

What happens to those who had hoped for a career in plastic surgery but were not capable of completing the requisite training? More often than not they transfer to other specialties where they find career fulfillment and success. But sometimes these doctors exploit an unwitting public (and a sizable regulatory loophole) to market themselves as plastic surgeons—which they are not.

Although it is hard to believe, there is no law preventing a gastroenterologist (whose specialty is the colon, intestines, and stomach) from performing plastic surgery if that doctor is certified as a physician. Of course this behavior is ethically questionable, but it is not illegal. Therefore patients must do their due diligence to protect themselves! This is especially important as the public becomes more willing to spend its own money on elective plastic surgery. With the burden of insurance paperwork growing exponentially and reimbursements dwindling, some doctors are tempted to cross over into plastic surgery (where most patients pay out-of-pocket), even if they are not qualified to do so.

In addition to the above regulatory loophole, there is also a big problem with the use of misleading language in how doctors present themselves to an unsuspecting public. More than any other medical specialty, there is an enormous amount of marketing hype in my field. This is due to the fact that most plastic surgery is both elective and inextricably bound to one's self-image. All of which conspires to make you, the patient, a very ripe target for unscrupulous sales pitches. The most egregious of these tactics is to use terms that have no meaning or weight in the medical community but that somehow imply experience and training that a doctor does not actually have.

This type of misleading advertising is everywhere and you need to know how to recognize it or else you may end up with a botched surgery. Let's say a gynecologist with no plastic surgery training wants to tap into the body-contouring market. You might read on his Web site that he is a board-certified physician (which he is). Then a few lines down you might see the terms *cosmetic surgeon* or *liposuction surgeon*. As these bits of information get processed you will probably end up with the misguided notion that this doctor is a board-certified plastic surgeon—which he is not.

In order to be certain you are dealing with a properly accredited plastic surgeon you should only consider a doctor who is a board-certified plastic surgeon—they are the real deal. In the medical community there is no such thing as a "cosmetic surgeon," so that term is a red flag someone is attempting to trick you. An ENT doctor can call himself a cosmetic surgeon and suffer no consequences, but he will face disciplinary action if he markets himself as a board-certified plastic surgeon. Many ENT doctors will call themselves "facial plastic surgeons" so that they can appear to be plastic surgeons. The American Board of Medical Specialties now recognizes facial plastic surgeon as a distinct entity, and there is nothing wrong with this label. But this certification entails less comprehensive training than plastic surgery does. So, while I have no doubt there are plenty of competent facial plastic surgeons out there, if I were you I would want a board-certified plastic surgeon doing my procedure. Then you are guaranteed to have a surgeon who has completed the most rigorous training in the field, end of story.

I find it both enraging and embarrassing that my fellow doctors would stoop to these levels to make a buck—and to put you at risk while doing so. But being upset about it does not make the hucksters go away, so the only thing I can do is educate you and hope that eventually this type of semantic sleight of hand no longer works.

To recap, you should only consider a board-certified plastic surgeon whose credentials are listed on the American Society of Plastic Surgeons' Web site, www.plasticsurgery.org. And while it is not absolutely necessary, I happen to believe a full residency in general surgery adds bonus points. Those five years of training can only increase a doctor's surgical know-how, improving his or her ability to problem solve while under pressure.

SHARED PHILOSOPHY

Because plastic surgery is usually elective—which means patients have a say in what is done—it is important to find a doctor who will approach and think about your issue in line with the way you do. Think of it a bit like house hunting. You have just looked at five properties that all fit within the same parameters—similar price, location, number of bedrooms, number of bathrooms—but you choose one over the others because it just "feels right." The same is true when selecting plastic surgeons. Once you have narrowed down your choices to properly trained and fully accredited doctors, it will be up to you to decide which one makes you feel most comfortable.

For example, I am somewhat wary of all the "new and improved" procedures that come and go every year (my philosophy is that new is not always better). If a patient of mine is interested in one of these procedures, I would present alternatives and use my medical expertise to explain why I think this particular surgery is a bad idea. However, there have been times when I have not been persuasive enough and the patient ultimately seeks out another doctor—one who will perform the surgery. This illustrates just one of the problems that can arise when a doctor and a patient do not share the same philosophy.

There are a lot of judgment calls made in plastic surgery: How much is enough? Are the benefits worth the trade-offs? Do I need surgery, or will a less-invasive procedure accomplish my goals? When is the right time for my procedure? You should find a doctor who is fundamentally in agreement with you on these matters of interpretation. In the end, you will be relying not just on her medical expertise to help you navigate this process, but also on her basic judgment as a person.

Of course, during a short consultation it may be hard to determine whether you two are a good fit for each other. My suggestion is to ask a few pointed questions about his or her approach and philosophy, after which you will probably have a solid understanding of your comfort level with this doctor. It is also not a bad idea to return for a second consultation after having had time to mull over what was discussed during the first meeting.

OFFICE TONE AND AMBIENCE

As a patient, you will be dealing with not only your surgeon but his or her staff as well. While it may sound trivial, the way the entire practice behaves toward you will affect your overall experience. You will find that a courteous and understanding staff is indispensable as you navigate territory that can be fraught with anxiety—about both your actual procedure as well as the "new you."

Doctors set the tone in their office; their concern, professionalism, and passion are usually mirrored by their staff members. Even the way someone answers the phone should be taken into consideration. A receptionist who is ornery or difficult could be a sign that the rest of the staff is the same—including the surgeon. And a responsive staff becomes especially critical during those rare times when something goes awry in surgery.

Because so much of plastic surgery relates to a patient's self-esteem, the level of emotional comfort you feel upon walking into your doctor's office really does matter. Upon finally finding the courage to speak to a professional about something you do not like about yourself, think of how devastated you would feel to be treated impersonally. Having made the big decision to undergo a procedure, it is so important to have a warm and supportive environment to rely upon throughout the process. You will not be too demanding if you expect that from your plastic surgeon's office.

"THE BEST"

I always find it amusing when patients assert that a particular plastic surgeon is "The Best." Just as it is hard to determine the best classical composer or Dutch master painter, the artistry of plastic surgery is equally difficult to quantify. There is no doubt that extensive technical training and a strong educational background are part of the equation. But there is an added element that transcends definition.

A truly gifted plastic surgeon—whatever his or her specialty may be—has a keen eye for balance and harmony like a fine painter does. This means fully appreciating the interdependent relationships and proportions of the problem area both before and after the surgery. If I take the painting metaphor a bit further, patients could be likened to a blank canvas upon arriving for a consultation. After listening to their issues and concerns, a plastic surgeon will begin to see what the finished "painting" should look like. And a really talented plastic surgeon will be able to translate that harmonious vision into reality.

Looking at "before" and "after" photos will help you determine a surgeon's ability to create and maintain the proper aesthetic balance. However, it is equally important to assess whether a doctor's suggestions make sense to you or not. Do they sound like appropriate solutions you would feel comfortable with? Or are they canned treatments that do not take into consideration your unique concerns? You may not be a surgeon, but you certainly know your face and body better than anyone else. Therefore, any suggestions need to feel right to you!

The lesson here is that there is no such thing as "the best" plastic surgeon. Instead, there are truly gifted surgeons who are only as good as their ability to address your needs in a balanced, appropriate, and successful manner.

EXPERIENCE

After you have narrowed down your search based on all of the above criteria, you will probably be left with a handful of specialists from which to choose. And this is where experience comes into play. A surgeon's experience can be measured in concrete terms: How long has he practiced? How many of a particular procedure has she performed? However, it is important to do your due diligence to cut through the hype.

With plastic surgeons now aggressively competing for your business, misleading claims can creep into marketing materials. I once came across a surgeon touting his skill with a particular procedure by claiming he had performed more than 10,000 of them! Upon doing the math—and knowing how long this surgeon had been in practice—I calculated he would have to be performing 30 of these procedures a week. Well, that simply strains credulity. But even if it were true, is that who you want doing your surgery? While this claim may support his experience, it does not say much about the level of personal attention you could expect to receive as a patient.

You want to find a surgeon who specializes in and has experience with the procedure you are considering. After meeting with him or her you should most definitely look at "before" and "after" photos that relate directly to the work you plan on having done. And, if at all possible, be allowed to speak to one or two former patients who have undergone the same procedure.

How much experience is enough? Just as few would eagerly volunteer to be a heart surgeon's first patient, it is understandable that not many would relish the idea of being a plastic surgeon's first facelift. But every surgeon in practice today did perform a first procedure on a patient, and more than likely it turned out fine. In twenty years' time would that surgeon look back and say, "That was my finest moment"? Probably not. But by the time plastic surgeons are in private practice, they have performed many, many procedures during their training. And that is why the rigor and competition of their educational training does matter—to ensure they are ready from day one.

As a young plastic surgeon I was knowledgeable and well trained, with a passion for the art of plastic surgery. But admittedly my experience was limited and my results were not as consistent as they are today. Having said that, experience is still somewhat difficult to define solely in terms of years. Some surgeons will be better right from the start, while others never make the grade despite years of training. As a rule, if a doctor satisfies all of your other criteria and has performed your procedure a significant number of times, then you should consider that surgeon sufficiently experienced.

PLASTIC SURGERY TOURISM

Recently there has been a growing and dangerous trend of Americans traveling abroad to save money on plastic surgery. There are myriad reasons to avoid this folly at all costs. Unless you are planning to stay for months after your surgery, there is a much greater risk that complications could develop because your recovery is not being properly monitored. If you have no postoperative care, what may have been a small problem could quickly turn into a serious one due to a delayed response. In my practice we consider postoperative care just as important as the actual surgery, and you should too. In addition, how can you possibly assess the quality of the surgeon—his or her training, accreditation, philosophy, and experience—if you are flying in the day before your surgery? If price were the only criteria when choosing a plastic surgeon, this chapter would have been considerably shorter! The old adage "you get what you pay for" rings true in this case. Don't look for a bargain when it comes to your body and well-being. In the end the cost may be too high.

Internet Resources: Plastic Surgery

    www.plasticsurgery.org/Patients_and_Consumers.html

    www.abms.org/Who_We_Help/Consumers/

Chapter 13

PREPARING FOR SURGERY

"Beauty lasts five minutes.
Maybe longer if you have good plastic surgeon."

—Tia Carrere

Deciding to have aesthetic surgery is a big step that should be taken only after much careful consideration. This becomes especially true when considering surgery on and around your face. Unlike a botched breast augmentation that might be more easily camouflaged, facial surgery "gone bad" is hard to hide and difficult to fix. Therefore, everyone involved—including you—needs to do his or her part to make sure it goes off without a hitch.

After reading this book you now have the skills to find the surgeon best suited for your particular needs, to assess which surgeries may (or may not) be appropriate for you, and to understand the pros and cons of each procedure. And with your surgery approaching, you may think it is time for your doctor to take over. While it is true that your surgeon will perform the procedure, the reality of the situation is that doctor-patient time together represents a very small proportion of the overall experience. You must be ready to assume responsibility for preparing yourself for a successful surgery, ensuring a speedy recovery, and avoiding any complications.

A MONTH BEFORE SURGERY

Communication is extremely important to any successful surgery. Make sure that all of your questions regarding the procedure have been answered by your doctor. It is best to do this well in advance—you do not need any unsettling surprises at the last minute. I often suggest to my patients that they have a small notebook where they can keep a running list of all of their questions and concerns. When they come in for their last consultation we use that as a point of reference to go over everything together. Believe it or not, it seems quite common for patients to meet their doctor only once, during the initial consultation, before seeing him on the way to the operating room. I feel strongly that this is no way for patients to understand the type of surgery they are choosing or to gain confidence in their surgeon. So make a point of meeting again with your doctor during the month leading up to your operation.

You should also provide your doctor with a list of all medications (both prescription and over the counter), herbal supplements, and vitamins you are taking. All of these chemicals enter the bloodstream, and some can negatively impact your surgery. This is especially important with herbal supplements. Because herbal medicines are not as widely used in the United States as in other parts of the world, many of the potential interactions are not completely understood here. Thus, you should vet these with your doctor well before your surgery.

This is the time to have all of your presurgical testing done. Your doctor will decide on the types of tests and clearances required to ensure that your body is in the proper condition to undertake the stresses of an elective cosmetic procedure. After testing, make sure that all results are forwarded to your plastic surgeon's office in a timely fashion—they don't help if they don't arrive!

Depending on your own set of family and work pressures, this is the moment you should start thinking about how to carve out the time needed to heal properly from your surgery. Recovery times vary depending on the procedure, but whether it is five days or two weeks, you must create a stress-free window for yourself or you run the risk of disrupting the critical healing process. Make sure to arrange all details such as child care, family schedules, and time off from work well in advance so you are not scrambling at the last minute.

A month before your surgery you should make a concerted effort to eat a nutritionally balanced diet high in protein, which supports the healing process. You should also supplement a healthy diet with three vitamins that are crucial to wound healing and blood clotting: A multivitamin, vitamin C ester, and vitamin K should be taken daily. A good multivitamin provides you with, among other things, daily doses of vitamin A and zinc, both of which promote proper healing. Vitamin C, which helps build collagen, is equally crucial to proper healing. I suggest the "ester" form of vitamin C because it is more easily absorbed by the body and so is more available for the healing process. Finally, vitamin K is important because it not only supports healing but also boosts blood clotting, which can help during and after surgery. I give my patients a prescription-strength form of vitamin K called Mephyton to begin taking two days before surgery.

It may come as a surprise to most readers that vitamin E, which is often associated with healing, should be avoided prior to surgery. While vitamin E oil can help heal the late stages of a scar (to be applied no sooner than two months after the surgery), taking vitamin E as a supplement prevents cross-collagen linkage, which can cause a scar to widen. In addition, vitamin E has been associated with an increased chance of bleeding. Needless to say, neither is desirable following a surgical procedure, so the vitamin should be avoided. Most multivitamins contain less than the limit of 400 IUs per day; ask your doctor to evaluate your multi to be sure.

Certain prescription drugs, such as MAO inhibitors Nardil and Parnate, should be avoided at least four weeks prior to surgery. These medications can interact with the anesthesia or pain medications and end with disastrous results. In order to wean your body off these medications properly and be given a safe alternative, you must see the doctor who prescribed them for you.

Remember that no matter how skilled your doctor is, any surgical procedure is a trauma to your body. The healthier you are, the better chance you have to heal safely and quickly after the procedure. A good diet, the proper supplements, close attention to a few caveats, and organizing a stress-free period around your surgery will ensure you do just that.

TWO WEEKS BEFORE SURGERY

As you get closer to your surgery, it becomes even more important to monitor what you put into your body. Again, this is especially true of any herbal supplements you may be taking. You must not take any supplements or homeopathic remedies that contain garlic, ginkgo biloba, ginger, Asian ginseng, or feverfew. These all slow blood coagulation by inhibiting the activity of platelets. In addition, any supplements that affect the skin (potentially causing an adverse reaction to the healing of your scar) must be avoided two weeks prior and two months after your surgery. These include St. John's wort, echinacea, melatonin, and aloe vera. A word of caution—if you are taking an herbal supplement that is not mentioned above I would still suggest you stop using it two weeks prior to surgery. My motto is "When in doubt, cut it out."

Finally, you should avoid all nonsteroidal anti-inflammatory pain medications as they, too, inhibit blood clotting and can lead to excessive bleeding during surgery. This means that pain relievers such as Advil, Aleve, Bufferin, Anacin, Excedrin, Motrin, naproxen sodium, Naprosyn, and all forms of aspirin must not be taken during this period—and this applies to some prescription analgesics as well. The only pain relief you should use is acetaminophen (Tylenol). If you need something stronger, consult with your surgeon. There are prescription narcotic pain medications that do not affect your blood's ability to clot.

This is the time to visit your pharmacy and get all of the prescriptions you will need for the surgery. Doing so well in advance allows for enough time to answer any questions you may have regarding your medications. When you pick up your prescriptions, be sure to read all of the instructions to make certain you understand them. And it is always a good idea to count the pills to confirm no mistakes have been made. You will be in no condition to correct even the slightest error immediately following your surgery, so it's best to do it now.

Finally, you should arrange for someone reliable to get you home after the surgery. Even if you feel okay and alert, you should absolutely not risk trying to get home on your own, even if it is just a matter of taking a cab by yourself. Anesthesia can affect people differently, and you might end up with nausea and vomiting as the anesthesia wears off. Needless to say, you do not want to face that possibility alone!

TWO DAYS BEFORE SURGERY

You should call your surgeon's office to confirm the details—including what to wear, what to bring, the time you should arrive, and the approximate time of the procedure. If anything seems different than what you were expecting, ask to speak with your doctor. Again, communication is key to a successful surgery, and this will be your last opportunity to ask a question, so do not be shy.

At this point you should avoid salty or spicy foods because these foods are associated with swelling, which is not a good thing right before surgery. You should also avoid these foods for at least one week following your surgery.

THE NIGHT BEFORE THE SURGERY

You will need to fast, which means that you cannot eat or drink anything after midnight on the evening prior to your surgery. The anesthesiologist will want your stomach completely empty of solids and liquids at the start of surgery to make sure that nothing can come back up during the surgery and get trapped in your lungs. Remember to take your supplements (multivitamin, vitamin C, and vitamin K) earlier in the day since you are not even allowed a small glass of water this close to surgery. You might want to put a note on the tap in case you are accustomed to waking up in the middle of the night for a drink of water.

Your anesthesiologist should telephone you the night before your surgery to go over the proper protocol—reminding you to fast, telling you about possible side effects, and answering any questions you may have. The purpose of this call is to help you stay informed while also reassuring you about the procedure.

THE DAY OF THE SURGERY

The time has come. All of your hard work—reading this book, searching for the right plastic surgeon, preparing properly for your procedure—is about to come to fruition. All of which is very exciting but also a bit unnerving, so expect to have some butterflies. Remember that you are going into surgery much better prepared than most people and, if you have followed the advice in this book, you should not be experiencing any last-minute doubts or worries.

Because you may suffer from dizziness after the procedure, wear flat shoes or sneakers. This way you will be in a better position to regain your balance if you feel faint or light-headed. Also, do not wear any cosmetics at all, including even a simple facial moisturizer. Some can contain metallic traces, which may interfere with the electronic equipment used in modern surgery. The same is true of jewelry, which you should not wear at all (even if the piece is worn away from the area to be worked on), as the metal can interfere with the electronic equipment and cause problems during the procedure. Remove nail polish from at least one finger of each hand. The device used to monitor your oxygen and heart rate must be fastened to a finger without nail polish. Finally, leave your contacts at home and wear your glasses instead.

You should bring all of your medications with you, especially if, after your procedure, you are planning to stay in a hotel or somewhere other than home for the night. The two most important medications to have readily available right after surgery are for pain and nausea. The most common postoperative complaints regard nausea from the anesthesia. Prevent this by taking one Zofran with a tiny sip of water two hours before the operation (remember, you will be fasting, so the sip must be very small). For patients who have a history of postoperative nausea I also prescribe a scopolamine patch, which is applied to the base of the neck 24 hours before surgery and stays there for two days.

AFTER YOUR SURGERY

When your surgery is over, your doctor's job is largely done. You will have a few additional appointments to check on your healing and to remove stitches, but most of the surgeon's work happens in the operating room. Now it is up to you.

Your first priority should be to follow all of your doctor's instructions to a T. I sometimes have patients who feel better than expected during the initial stages of their recovery so they start to jump ahead of my recommendations. This is really not a good idea because your body requires time to recover and heal properly. You risk doing damage to the end results of your surgery by not following your doctor's instructions. I also give patients my cell phone number, encouraging them to call with any questions they may have, regardless of how insignificant they may seem. I have found that, for the most part, patients do not abuse this privilege and call with appropriate questions and concerns that aid in a better recovery.

I will not sugarcoat the fact that you should expect some discomfort the first few days following your surgery. Of course, this will depend on the particular procedure you have undergone, but more than likely you will experience varying degrees of pain afterward. You will probably be prescribed a painkiller such as Vicodin or Percocet. Remember that these are narcotics and can become addictive, so approach them with care. Once your pain subsides you should stop taking the pills, even if you have not finished your prescription. Also, you must not take aspirin for at least 10 days following your surgery.

To ward off infection, your doctor will also prescribe an antibiotic. Unlike the pain medication, you must finish all of your antibiotic pills and be sure to take them at the prescribed times. If not, they become ineffective. And the last thing you want at the end of this long process is an infection!

It is critical to take proper care of your wounds and eventual scars. The skill of your plastic surgeon is important in determining the quality of your scars, but so is the aftercare. Follow these guidelines to improve the eventual outcome at the incision area:

Listen to everything your physician tells you regarding the care of your wound. During the first two weeks the healing incision is very weak and prone to widening and disruption. Therefore, you must limit any activity that could put stress or tension on the incision.

Continue with the vitamin C ester. This will help the maturing wound establish the proper amount and quality of collagen that is necessary to build strong, healthy tissue.

After the stitches are removed, **ask your doctor about anti-scar creams, gels, and sheets.** I recommend silicone gel sheets or pads applied to the wound 12 hours a day for the first six weeks. Neosporin brand silicone sheeting is available at your local pharmacy and works fine. Keep in mind that every sheet is reusable.

Avoid topical steroid creams! Steroids can make the scar thin out and widen. Beware that in the drugstore next to the silicone sheeting are products that have silicone as well as a steroid (usually hydrocortisone). Stay away from these products.

If you have any scabs on the incision after the stitches have been removed, I suggest **frequent application (four or five times per day) of Bacitracin or Neosporin** until the scab goes away. Of course, if the wound starts to look abnormal, consult with your surgeon.

Avoid the sun at the incision site for six months after the procedure. The ultraviolet rays will change the color of the incision, making it lighter (in light-skinned individuals) or darker (in dark-skinned individuals). Remember that UVA rays can penetrate clothing, so apply the proper sunscreen and reapply it often (see chapter 4).

For patients whose scars begin to turn bright red or become raised and hard, you should **ask your doctor about specific laser treatments** that may help eliminate or soften these scars. You should not consider any of these treatments until four to six weeks after the procedure.

	Wound Care	Downtime in Weeks			Other Considerations
		Out in Public	Light Exercise	Heavy Exercise	
Facelift	Bacitracin to incision sites; cold compresses are on for 24 hrs.; dressings for 1–3 days; stitches are removed 1 week after surgery	2	3	4	skin is numb on the cheeks for 3–6 months
Neck Lift	same as facelift	1	2	3	–
Rhino-plasty	cold compresses for 24 hours; cast on nose for 1 week	1	3	6	humidify bedroom for added comfort
Blepharo-plasty	cold compresses for 24 hours; no dressings; eye lubrication is a must; sutures are removed 4–5 days after surgery	1–2	3	3	do eye exercises after the stitches come out to reduce swelling
Brow Lift	cold compresses on the forehead; no dressings; sutures out in 14 days	3–4	3	3	forehead numbness may last for 6 months
Otoplasty	headdress for 1–2 weeks, followed by sweatband over ears for an additional month	when dressing comes off	6	6	stay away from anyone trying to play with ears

Chapter 14

TEENS AND COSMETIC SURGERY

"If there is one thing worse than being an ugly duckling in a house of swans, it's having the swans pretend there's no difference."

—Teena Booth

T hroughout this book I have emphasized the need for patients to be aware of the psychological as well as the physical implications of cosmetic surgery. These psychological components become even more critical when the patient is a teenager. Since plastic surgery alters the way you look and is so intrinsically bound to your self-esteem, a certain level of emotional maturity is necessary. With adult patients I can usually assume that the decision to undergo plastic surgery has been made rationally. Not so with teens, who may not have the maturity required to temper rash impulses driven by a beauty-obsessed culture. Today's teens are bombarded with images of celebrities their own age who have the perfect smile, the perfect body, and the perfect nose, making almost anyone else feel imperfect in comparison.

A few years back I was approached by a TV producer who was looking for plastic surgeons to perform teen makeovers on a reality show. The premise was that these teenagers could pick their favorite teen celebrity and be made to look like that person through the use of surgical procedures. After getting over my initial shock that anyone could be peddling this as entertainment, I made it clear that I would not be involved while also weighing in on how dangerous and exploitative the show's premise was. Well, I suppose it says a lot about current societal mores that the show eventually became a hit. I mention this not only because I was outraged. It is also a perfect example of how media-driven messaging makes it so difficult for parents to help teenagers sort through the complicated question of whether plastic surgery is appropriate for them or not.

This chapter offers parents guidelines to help do just that in an emotionally sensitive and logical manner. Of course, because teens mature differently, each case is unique and there are always exceptions to rules. But by following these guidelines you will be able to judge whether your teen is a viable enough candidate to even take the step of meeting with a plastic surgeon. And by educating yourself on the topic you will be providing your child with what he or she needs most—a level-headed parent committed to operating in his or her child's best interest.

It should be pointed out, before I go any further, that parents should never suggest plastic surgery to their teenager. This is bound to create problems even if it is done with good intentions. I have had plenty of adult patients who, after experiencing a successful surgery, will confide in me that they think their teen needs a nose job or his ears fixed. Parents will go to any length to protect their children, so I understand and appreciate this impulse to "fix" something. However, I strongly urge parents not to say anything. They should wait for the teen to broach the subject himself. The developing self-esteem of an adolescent is fragile and can be badly damaged if a parent is perceived as pointing out a shortcoming. And if your child is not concerned about her "imperfection," then more than likely you should not be either. The last thing you want to do is give your child a complex when none existed. However, if you honestly believe surgery is in the best interest of your teen's emotional health (and you sense he may be too ashamed to speak about it), there are indirect ways to encourage a discussion. For example, while watching TV or flipping through a tabloid magazine you could start a neutral conversation about a celebrity's plastic surgery and see what your teen has to say about it. This might be the opening she was waiting for. Just remember that whenever you discuss your child's physical features you should choose your words very carefully, as your opinion will have a big impact on the way he sees himself.

ASSESSING THE SITUATION

Assuming that your child comes to you, asking about plastic surgery, the first thing you, as the parent, should do is determine how real the need for surgery is. You are not a doctor and thus are not capable of making a medical assessment. However, you know your child better than any doctor, so it will initially be up to you to gauge if the desire for surgery is legitimate. Is the problem pronounced enough that your teenager is being teased by other kids? Would the correction of the physical deformity be enough to return that child's life to normalcy? Is the imperfection something you yourself had been aware of and worried about, too?

The above questions should be relatively straightforward to answer. The real challenge is in getting a clear idea of what the teen's expectations are, determining whether peer pressure has been an influencing factor, and understanding what the underlying motivation for suddenly wanting the surgery is.

EXPECTATIONS

Once you have determined that your child has a legitimate need for corrective surgery, it is important to have a frank discussion with her about her expectations and what she hopes to gain from the procedure. Teens who believe that they will become the most popular student in school or will suddenly start dating the star quarterback because the bump on their nose has been fixed are not ready for plastic surgery. You must make it clear to your teenager that there is no such thing as a magic bullet, capable of erasing the standard angst and woes that are part of growing up. Any teen who thinks that a particular procedure will offer that type of transformation has unrealistic expectations and, again, is not yet emotionally mature enough to be a patient. The best place to start any discussion on this topic is asking your teenager: "How do you think your life will change once the problem is corrected?" It is your responsibility, as the adult, to listen very carefully to the answer.

PEER PRESSURE

Teens, probably more than any other age group, are particularly susceptible to what their friends think, and they modify their behavior to conform. Taken to an extreme, peer pressure can now include the option to surgically alter yourself to be "normal" and to fit in more easily. If all of your daughter's friends have small noses and she doesn't, she may feel pressure to look more like her peers. So it is important to understand why your child wants a particular procedure. This becomes especially true if you have never noticed the "deformity" that is suddenly the focus of her attention. Being the target of merciless teasing for ears that stick out is one thing. Your daughter feeling like she doesn't quite fit in because of a slightly larger nose is quite another. It will be up to you to assess how legitimate your child's need for surgery is.

MOTIVATION

The final factor in gauging whether your child is a viable candidate for plastic surgery is in understanding what is motivating her or him to consider surgery. The best way to determine this is to ask a few questions, the first of which should be, "How long has this problem bothered you?" If it turns out that your teen has struggled with the issue for a long time and is finally requesting corrective surgery, this might be a sign of a growing level of maturity. Another question to ask is, "Why do you want the surgery now?" If your teen presents logical reasons for the timing, then this, too, could be confirmation that he has the necessary maturity level. However, be wary of any motivating factor that sounds like your teen is choosing the easy way out. Adolescence is a difficult time and, unfortunately, a little bit of teasing tends to be part of growing up. You will need to decide whether or not your teen should tough it out for a few more years—and learn some valuable life lessons in the process.

There are some groups of teens who should never undergo plastic surgery. Any teenager who is currently battling depression, drug addition, bulimia, or anorexia is not a viable candidate and should seek psychological help for those problems. In addition, if your teen seems obsessed with having plastic surgery despite everyone's assurances that she is attractive, she may be suffering from a psychological disorder called body dysmorphic disorder (BDD). Experts believe that as many as five million people in the United Sates suffer from BDD and that the most common time of onset is during adolescence. BDD is characterized by obsessive unhappiness with a particular body part. People suffering from BDD may hate their nose, lips, or ears, even if there is absolutely nothing wrong with them. Of course, it then follows that the slightest actual deformity becomes a complete obsession of the BDD sufferer. Those suffering from BDD believe that not only are they aware of and consumed by their (perceived) disfigurement, but that everyone else is as well. Clinical research has shown that in almost all cases cosmetic surgery does nothing to improve BDD sufferers' satisfaction with their features. If it sounds like this may be your teen's problem, plastic surgery is not a viable option and, instead, you should seek help from a professional therapist.

MEDICAL CONSULTATION

Once you have come to the conclusion that your teenager is a legitimate candidate for corrective surgery and possesses enough emotional maturity to handle it, you should make a consultation appointment with a plastic surgeon (see chapter 12). It will be up to the plastic surgeon to assess both the physical and the emotional maturity of your teenager to determine which, if any, surgical options are available. This is also the time for your teen to be told, in very clear language, the pros and cons of the procedure,

not only gives an impression of youth, but remaining optimistic and upbeat as you get older helps your skin stay younger looking. Negativity, pessimism, and cynicism only cause more worry lines, more wrinkles, and the production of damaging free radicals. So putting on a "happy face" is not only more pleasant for the people around you—it is healthier for your skin and your body!

SLEEP

It is very hard to look your best when you are tired. Lack of sleep is not only immediately apparent, but it also ends up causing cumulative damage to your skin. If you are not getting enough sleep due to stress or other factors, your body produces extra cortisol, which can retard skin regeneration during the nighttime hours when regeneration should be at its highest. It follows logically that if you are not getting enough sleep, preventing your skin from regenerating properly, you are going to look older.

DIET

Eating a nutritionally balanced diet of natural and unprocessed foods is very important to staying young-looking. But since current information on nutrition and diet is so confusing, it is sometimes difficult to know what to do. I always tell my patients that the two most important fundamentals of healthy eating habits are common sense and moderation.

Earlier humans were grazers, eating on and off throughout the day when food became available. While societal habits have changed, our bodies have not. After about three and a half hours of not eating our systems kick into "starvation mode," which means that calories ingested during that time are stored—usually as fat—for protection against famine. Because of this mechanism, it would logically follow that one of the simpler ways of avoiding fat storage is to minimize the number of times your body goes into starvation mode. Obviously, you are not going to wake up in the middle of the night to eat a protein bar. But keep in mind that breakfast should be your only meal when your body is in starvation mode. (Eating carbohydrates in the morning—as so many people do—ensures that these calories will end up stored as fat. Protein, on the other hand, does not get converted into fat, which is why an egg breakfast is a good idea.) I should be clear that the recommendation to eat every three and a half hours does not give you license to enjoy a large, sit-down meal five times a day. Rather, a slice of cheese or a handful of nuts (both rich in protein, you will note) are effective in keeping your body out of starvation mode and your blood sugar stable.

The success of any healthy diet depends on moderation. This means not denying yourself one particular food group or going overboard on others. Studies show that most diets based on deprivation or a limited selection end up becoming counterproductive in the long run. Low-carb diets are a perfect example of this cycle. Yes, you may lose weight the first few months. But then what happens when you are at your goal weight and want a piece of bread? It is not hard to understand the psychological impact of cutting out an entire food group from your diet—it only makes you want it more. And that is not a recipe for long-term success.

Be aware of the nutritional value of the food that you eat. I often tell my patients to avoid white foods. While that may sound like an oversimplification (which it is), for those of us who are not professional nutritionists it is an easy rule to follow that certainly cannot hurt. For example, instead of white bread or white rice opt for whole wheat bread or brown rice. Remember that processing food diminishes its nutritional benefits, so any food is better for you when it is closest to its most natural state. Substitute saturated fats with healthier ones such as olive oil, which is great for both cooking and drizzling on bread instead of butter.

Drink lots of water. Keeping your skin hydrated is key to keeping it young-looking.

Eat food slowly and with awareness. There is a time lag of at least 15 minutes for your brain to understand that you have eaten to your full capacity. Thus, eating quickly can often result in eating too much. If you are lucky enough to be dining with others, slow down and enjoy some conversation (although not with your mouth full!). If you are eating alone it becomes even more important to guard against wolfing down your meal too fast. So take your time and savor each bite—even if it is just a frozen entrée you are eating in front of the TV.

Take supplements to make sure that you are getting the recommended daily dosage of the vitamins and minerals that you need. It is always best to eat healthy foods rich in vitamins, but sometimes it does not always work out that way. Therefore, supplementing your diet with vitamins (most especially antioxidants that neutralize damaging free radicals) is very important to your overall health—including that of your skin!

The "Beauty Food" regimen described in appendix A is designed not as a diet, or a way to deny you the foods you crave, but as a guideline of simple foods that will provide the designed nutritional elements that are necessary to ward off Father Time and Mother Nature at the same time. So look it over and use the parts that feel comfortable to your lifestyle and eating habits.

EXERCISE

Staying active and maintaining a certain level of fitness is very important to your long-term health. It also goes a long way in keeping you vibrant and looking young. Whether it is a daily walk, regular sessions at the gym, or your weekly tennis game, the first goal is to keep moving. This strategy will not only be good for your heart but will also be great for your attitude—regular exercise can only make you feel better about yourself. Keep in mind that if weight loss is your goal and your time is limited you should choose muscle-developing activities (squats, lunges, ab crunches) over aerobic exercise (walking, running, biking) because increased muscle tone burns more calories. For example, if you work out on the treadmill and burn 350 calories, the moment you step off the machine the calorie-burning benefit of that workout ends. However, if you spent the same amount of time doing lunges or squats for a month, the amount of calories burned from that activity would be higher because those newly developed muscles continue to burn calories even while resting. What's more, the bigger the muscle, the more calories it burns. Therefore, a really toned thigh or butt will be extremely effective in getting rid of excess calories. Finally, try to find an exercise routine that you actually enjoy—that way, you will be more apt to do it regularly.

SKIN CARE

As you have already learned in chapter 4, over-the-counter products can accomplish only so much in keeping your skin young-looking. Therefore, I do recommend that you visit a dermatologist to get started on a more effective skin care regimen. Regular skin maintenance includes a mild cleanser, an antioxidant moisturizer, and a good sunblock (used in that order), as well as exfoliating at least once a week. In addition to these basics, you should speak to your dermatologist about either a Retin-A or an AHA cream to be applied in the evening (remember that both will make your skin more sensitive to the sun). These can help regenerate your skin on the cellular level. If, after following the above regimen for a while, you feel your skin needs more of a "boost," you might consider one of the more invasive cosmetic procedures such as peels, fillers, or Botox (outlined in chapter 3). But please remember that the dermatologist is not just there to rejuvenate your skin—an annual visit is critical in your fight against any type of skin cancer.

Beyond the doctor's office, there are lifestyle choices that greatly affect the quality of your skin, and I consider these to be "skin care" as well. Drinking alcohol in excess and smoking cigarettes not only damage your skin but also degrade its ability to regenerate properly after that damage. Environmental factors are also important elements of your overall skin care. Try to keep your house humidified and toxin/pollutant free. Finally, as silly as it may sound, using a satin pillowcase and sleeping on your back put less stress on the skin of your face, so both are good habits to incorporate into your life.

DENTAL CARE

Regular visits to the dentist will help ensure that your teeth look good and remain healthy. This is important because healthy teeth and gums keep your face young-looking by maintaining its shape and proportion. Beyond cleanings twice a year, you might also consider an in-office whitening treatment that can perk up your looks a bit. And if you have any problems with cracked or crooked teeth, you should most definitely take care of these sooner rather than later. Healthy teeth is not just a matter of aesthetics—ignoring small issues now can cause serious structural problems in the future that can change your entire face. And, of course, brush twice a day, floss once a day, and use a fluoride mouthwash to guard against gingivitis and tooth decay. These are all rather easy, small steps to take to ensure healthy teeth for as long as you live.

WARDROBE UPDATE

Yes, it is true—I am suggesting that you buy new clothes! And if that is the only reason you would actually go out and shop for some new outfits, then you are probably a prime candidate for a makeover. While some may consider what you wear to be a superficial consideration, I disagree. The way you dress says a lot about who you are and how you feel about yourself; take care to manage that message as well as you can. Think of how great you feel when attending a special event in an elegant outfit. Of course, none of us can walk around in black-tie clothes every day. My point is that taking care of what you wear (while staying age and body appropriate) acts as a real boost to your self-image and allows you to project a positive attitude. If you have the money to spend I would suggest going to a wardrobe consultant at one of the major department stores. If that is out of reach, why not ask a friend or relative who is particularly sharp to help you find the best clothes that maximize your potential? And don't be afraid even if it means trying new things. Experimenting with the persona you project to the world can only help in finding the best look for you.

HAIR CARE

In addition to keeping your hair healthy and attractive (see chapters 5 and 11), there are a number of ways to update your look by visiting the hair salon. Most stylists will offer a complimentary consultation. It cannot hurt to at least hear some new ideas regarding your cut, style, and color. I find that most people fall into a rut with their hair and stick with the status quo only because no one has suggested otherwise. It is amazing how rejuvenated a face can look by just manipulating the hair around it, so do not be shy about experimenting a bit. Remember, hair grows back. And the boost to your self-esteem from making these changes can only add to your positive attitude. All of which translates to a younger looking you!

MAKEUP

Most women fall into the "status quo" rut with their makeup as well. I consider it money well spent to seek out the professional opinion of a makeup consultant. If that is not financially feasible, you can visit the cosmetics counter at a high-end depart-ment store to receive some guidance about application as well as new products on the market. In one hour, a pro can teach you "tricks" that have the potential to benefit you for the rest of your life. And, just like clothes, your makeup (or lack thereof) does tell people something about you. So take the time to find the right look for you and use it to project your best face forward.

PLASTIC SURGERY

I would encourage anyone considering a procedure to set up an initial consultation with a plastic surgeon. After reading this book, you should be informed enough to make the most of that first meeting. You should go to that consultation knowing what you are interested in having done rather than asking the doctor to make that call for you. To prepare for the consultation, please refer to the chapter in this book that relates to your area of concern and review chapter 12 regarding how to find a surgeon best suited for you. You will also want to compile a list of questions and concerns you have regarding any potential procedures—this way, you walk away from that first meeting with as much information as possible.

Just remember that, in the end, beauty emanates from the inside out. So any habit you can embrace, any product you can buy, any regimen you can implement that helps you feel more positive about life—and yourself—will lead the way to a more beautiful you.

BEAUTY FOOD

Y ou may be asking yourself, "What is a diet doing in a beauty book?" Vitamin regimens and antioxidants are the latest overhyped ways to look and feel younger, but it is possible to consume your nutrients through a natural regimen of healthy foods instead of costly supplements. Most diets fail as a result of deprivation and the desire to have something that is forbidden. "Beauty Food" is not a diet, but a guide to some great foods that are easily made and tasty and certainly will help enhance your outer and inner beauty.

I know that taking the information outlined in this book and putting it into practice can be a daunting task. So, along with the Diet Diva, Keri Gans, I have developed an eating regimen that will encompass all of the nutrients, vitamins, and minerals essential to preserving healthy, youthful skin. Note that I have not specified beverages, but they are no less important. Drink plenty of water on a daily basis—at least eight glasses per day. Drinking one or two glasses of red wine a day is good for the antioxidant effects and high dose of resveratrol. Avoid caffeinated drinks; if you are a coffee lover, stick with decaf. As for soda, I remember some time ago having a carbonated cola stain on my car that ate away at the paint job. These sugary or artificial sweetened drinks are not great for your body, either, so when you are trying to look your best, stick with water.

Now "Beauty Food" is not a promise of the fountain of youth, nor will it transform you into a Hollywood starlet. Our goals are much more modest ones—fight the fight against Father Time and slow the process of aging.

DAY 1

Breakfast

Oatmeal

    (½ cup oats, 1 cup skim milk, 1 tablespoon
    ground flaxseed, sprinkle cinnamon)

1 cup strawberries

Snack

Whole-grain crispbread with
1 tablespoon natural peanut butter

Lunch

Chicken sandwich

    (2 slices whole wheat bread, 3 ounces grilled
    chicken, 1 tablespoon hummus, lettuce,
    tomato)

Snack

½ cup low-fat plain yogurt

1 cup melon

Dinner

3 ounces grilled salmon, sautéed in
2 teaspoons olive oil

1 cup steamed broccoli

½ cup quinoa

Mixed green salad with ½ cup tomatoes, salad
dressing spray, 1 tablespoon ground flaxseed

Snack

Orange

nutrition breakdown	grams	calories	% total
Fat	47	423	24
Carbs	260	868	50
Fiber	43	0	0
Protein	112	448	26
Total		1739	

fat-soluble vitamins	intake	RDA	% RDA
Vitamin A	1086.8 mg	800 mg	136
Vitamin D	2.45 IU	5	49
		IU	
Vitamin E	9.47 mg	8 mg	118
Vitamin K	197.95 mcg	65 mcg	305

trace minerals	intake	RDA	% RDA
Iron	15.78 mg	15 mg	105
Zinc	10.81 mg	12 mg	90
Selenium	111.02 mcg	55 mcg	202
Copper	1.59 mg	—	—

water-soluble vitamins	intake	RDA	% RDA
Vitamin C	346.46 mg	60 mg	577
Thiamin	1.66 mg	1.1 mg	151
Riboflavin	1.58 mg	1.1 mg	143
Vitamin B6	1.96 mg	1.3 mg	150
Vitamin B12	4.62 mcg	2.4 mcg	192
Niacin	25.23 mg	14 mg	180
Folate	498.8 mcg	400 mcg	125

major minerals	intake	RDA	% RDA
Calcium	923.18 mg	1000 mg	92
Phosphorus	1762.8 mg	700 mg	252
Magnesium	507.01 mg	310 mg	164
Sodium	1624.8 mg	—	—
Potassium	3738 mg	—	—

	intake	RDA	% AI
Omega-3	5.387 g	1.6 g	336.7

	grams	calories	% total
nutrition breakdown			
Fat	52	468	28
Carbs	220	700	42
Fiber	45	0	0
Protein	125	500	30
Total		1668	

	intake	RDA	% RDA
fat-soluble vitamins			
Vitamin A	4130.4 mg	800 mg	516
Vitamin D	0 IU	5 IU	0
Vitamin E	13.1 mg	8 mg	164
Vitamin K	195.99 mcg	65 mcg	302

	intake	RDA	% RDA
trace minerals			
Iron	14.44 mg	15 mg	96
Zinc	10.17 mg	12 mg	85
Selenium	177.27 mcg	55 mcg	322
Copper	1.52 mg	—	—

	intake	RDA	% RDA
water-soluble vitamins			
Vitamin C	206.39 mg	60 mg	344
Thiamin	1.02 mg	1.1 mg	93
Riboflavin	1.66 mg	1.1 mg	151
Vitamin B6	2.51 mg	1.3 mg	193
Vitamin B12	6.79 mcg	2.4 mcg	283
Niacin	41.53 mg	14 mg	297
Folate	681.72 mcg	400 mcg	170

	intake	RDA	% RDA
major minerals			
Calcium	1042.4 mg	1000 mg	104
Phosphorus	1508.8 mg	700 mg	216
Magnesium	411.42 mg	310 mg	1333
Sodium	3246.9 mg	—	—
Potassium	3373 mg	—	—

	intake	RDA	% AI
Omega-3	2.36 g	1.6 g	148

Breakfast

1 cup plain nonfat yogurt with 1 cup blueberries,
1 cup whole grain, high-fiber cereal,
1 tablespoon ground flaxseed

Snack

1 ounce almonds

Lunch

Tuna wrap

> (whole wheat wrap, individual can tuna packed in water, 1 tablespoon lowfat mayo, lettuce, cucumber, tomato)

1 cup vegetarian split pea soup

Snack

Medium apple

String cheese

Dinner

3 ounces grilled chicken drizzled with balsamic vinegar and rosemary

Medium sweet potato

Grilled asparagus (14 small spears), cooked in 2 teaspoons olive oil

Mixed green salad with ½ cup tomatoes, ¼ cup chickpeas, ½ cup cremini mushrooms, 1 tablespoon ground flaxseed, salad dressing spray

Snack

1 cup strawberries with
1 tablespoon whipped cream

Breakfast

Scrambled eggs (3 whites and 1 yolk)
with ½ cup tomatoes

2 slices whole wheat toast with
1 tablespoon low-fat cream cheese

Snack

1 cup low-fat cottage cheese with 1 cup berries
and 1 tablespoon ground flaxseed

Lunch

Mixed green salad with 3 ounces grilled chicken,
½ cup chickpeas, ½ cup beets, ½ cup artichoke
hearts, ½ cup shredded carrots, 1 tablespoon
ground flaxseed

Small whole grain roll

Snack

Pear with 1 tablespoon natural almond butter

Dinner

1 cup brown rice

8 large scallops sautéed in 2 teaspoons olive oil

1 cup Swiss chard

Snack

Baked apple with 2 tablespoons
nonfat plain yogurt

nutrition breakdown	grams	calories	% total
Fat	51	459	27
Carbs	233	728	43
Fiber	51	0	0
Protein	128	512	30
Total		1699	

fat-soluble vitamins	intake	RDA	% RDA
Vitamin A	2708.9 mg	800 mg	339
Vitamin D	0.626 IU	5 IU	13
Vitamin E	16.78 mg	8 mg	210
Vitamin K	199.92 mcg	65 mcg	308

trace minerals	intake	RDA	% RDA
Iron	17.8 mg	15 mg	119
Zinc	11.6 mg	12 mg	97
Selenium	165.3 mcg	55 mcg	301
Copper	1.95 mg	—	—

water-soluble vitamins	intake	RDA	% RDA
Vitamin C	134.9 mg	60 mg	225
Thiamin	1.09 mg	1.1 mg	99
Riboflavin	2.15 mg	1.1 mg	196
Vitamin B6	2.67 mg	1.3 mg	205
Vitamin B12	4.55 mcg	2.4 mcg	190
Niacin	24.31 mg	14 mg	174
Folate	537.5 mcg	400 mcg	134

major minerals	intake	RDA	% RDA
Calcium	773 mg	1000 mg	77
Phosphorus	1794 mg	700 mg	256
Magnesium	669 mg	310 mg	216
Sodium	3623 mg	—	—
Potassium	4310 mg	—	—

	intake	RDA	% AI
Omega-3	2.225 g	1.6 g	139

	grams	calories	% total
nutrition breakdown			
Fat	56	504	30
Carbs	217	700	42
Fiber	42	0	0
Protein	117	468	28
Total		1672	

	intake	RDA	% RDA
fat-soluble vitamins			
Vitamin A	2263.1 mg	800 mg	283
Vitamin D	4.97 IU	5 IU	99
Vitamin E	7.89 mg	8 mg	99
Vitamin K	197.1 mcg	65 mcg	303

	intake	RDA	% RDA
trace minerals			
Iron	14.5 mg	15 mg	97
Zinc	13.56 mg	12 mg	113
Selenium	93.92 mcg	55 mcg	171
Copper	1.98 mg	—	—

	intake	RDA	% RDA
water-soluble vitamins			
Vitamin C	224.18 mg	60 mg	374
Thiamin	1.77 mg	1.1 mg	161
Riboflavin	1.91 mg	1.1 mg	173
Vitamin B6	1.95 mg	1.3 mg	150
Vitamin B12	18.59 mcg	2.4 mcg	775
Niacin	20.23 mg	14 mg	145
Folate	500.48 mcg	400 mcg	125

	intake	RDA	% RDA
major minerals			
Calcium	1102.8 mg	1000 mg	110
Phosphorus	1882.6 mg	700 mg	269
Magnesium	517.51 mg	310 mg	167
Sodium	2262.9 mg	—	—
Potassium	4003.7 mg	—	—

	intake	RDA	% AI
Omega-3	4.207 g	1.6 g	263

Breakfast

Oatmeal

(½ cup oats, 1 cup skim milk, ½ cup blueberries, ½ ounce crushed walnuts, 1 tablespoon ground flaxseed, sprinkle cinnamon)

Snack

½ cup low-fat plain yogurt

½ cup blueberries

Lunch

Veggie burger on a whole wheat English muffin with 1 tablespoon hummus, lettuce, tomato

Medium orange

Snack

Whole grain crispbread with an individual can of water-packed sardines

Dinner

Large mixed green salad with ½ cup tomatoes, ½ cup carrots, ½ cup yellow peppers, salad dressing spray, 1 tablespoon ground flaxseed

3 ounces grilled sirloin steak

¾ cup whole wheat couscous

Roasted Brussels sprouts, spritzed with 1 teaspoon olive oil

Snack

1 cup cherries

DAY 5

Breakfast

Whole wheat wrap with 3 scrambled egg whites,
1 tablespoon low-fat cream cheese, 1 cup
spinach, 1 ounce feta cheese

Half a grapefruit

Snack

Small banana with 1 cup low-fat cottage cheese

Lunch

Large mixed green salad with 3 ounces grilled
chicken breast, ½ cup cucumber, ½ cup
carrots, ½ cup tomatoes, ½ cup apple slices,
1 tablespoon ground flaxseed

Small whole grain roll

Snack

Medium pear

1 ounce pumpkin seeds

Dinner

Pasta with shrimp, white beans, and broccoli rabe
(made with 1 cup whole wheat pasta, ½ cup
Great Northern beans, 8 medium-size grilled
shrimp, 2 teaspoons olive oil, ½ cup tomatoes,
1 cup broccoli rabe)

Mixed green salad with ½ cup beets, 1 tablespoon
ground flaxseed, salad dressing spray

Snack

3 cups air-popped popcorn

nutrition breakdown	grams	calories	% total
Fat	57	513	29
Carbs	238	768	43
Fiber	46	0	0
Protein	128	512	29
Total		1793	

fat-soluble vitamins	intake	RDA	% RDA
Vitamin A	3095.8 mg	800 mg	387
Vitamin D	1.98 IU	5 IU	40
Vitamin E	8.48 mg	8 mg	106
Vitamin K	418.04 mcg	65 mcg	643

trace minerals	intake	RDA	% RDA
Iron	18.52 mg	15 mg	123
Zinc	10.41 mg	12 mg	87
Selenium	112.0 mcg	55 mcg	204
Copper	2.02 mg	—	—

water-soluble vitamins	intake	RDA	% RDA
Vitamin C	177.45 mg	60 mg	296
Thiamin	1.02 mg	1.1 mg	93
Riboflavin	2.06 mg	1.1 mg	187
Vitamin B6	2.33 mg	1.3 mg	179
Vitamin B12	2.69 mcg	2.4 mcg	112
Niacin	15.6 mg	14 mg	111
Folate	660.96 mcg	400 mcg	165

major minerals	intake	RDA	% RDA
Calcium	798.4 mg	1000 mg	80
Phosphorus	1634.5 mg	700 mg	233
Magnesium	593 mg	310 mg	191
Sodium	2854.3 mg	—	—
Potassium	4033.3 mg	—	—

	intake	RDA	% AI
Omega-3	1.825 g	1.6 g	114

nutrition breakdown	grams	calories	% total
Fat	50	450	26
Carbs	238	768	44
Fiber	46	0	0
Protein	133	532	30
Total		1750	

fat-soluble vitamins	intake	RDA	% RDA
Vitamin A	1071.9 mg	800 mg	134
Vitamin D	0 IU	5 IU	0
Vitamin E	7.03 mg	8 mg	88
Vitamin K	206.33 mcg	65 mcg	317

trace minerals	intake	RDA	% RDA
Iron	15.76 mg	15 mg	105
Zinc	14.47 mg	12 mg	121
Selenium	132.05 mcg	55 mcg	240
Copper	2.05 mg	—	—

water-soluble vitamins	intake	RDA	% RDA
Vitamin C	263.56 mg	60 mg	439
Thiamin	1.23 mg	1.1 mg	112
Riboflavin	2.1 mg	1.1 mg	191
Vitamin B6	2.89 mg	1.3 mg	222
Vitamin B12	4.18 mcg	2.4 mcg	174
Niacin	24.42 mg	14 mg	174
Folate	644.67 mcg	400 mcg	161

major minerals	intake	RDA	% RDA
Calcium	1026.3 mg	1000 mg	103
Phosphorus	2037.6 mg	700 mg	291
Magnesium	627.35 mg	310 mg	202
Sodium	2759.2 mg	—	—
Potassium	4666.3 mg	—	—

	intake	RDA	% AI
Omega-3	4.20 g	1.6 g	262

Breakfast

1 cup plain, low-fat yogurt with 1 cup strawberries,
1 cup whole grain, high-fiber cereal,
1 tablespoon ground flaxseed

Snack

Whole grain crispbread with 1 tablespoon natural peanut butter

Lunch

Turkey-avocado sandwich

(2 slices whole wheat bread, 3 ounces turkey,
⅛ avocado, lettuce, tomato, Dijon mustard)

1 cup cantaloupe

Snack

1 cup low-fat cottage cheese

1 ounce soy nuts

Dinner

Mixed green salad with ½ cup chickpeas,
½ cup tomatoes, 1 tablespoon ground flaxseed,
salad dressing spritzer

3 ounces halibut

1 cup wild rice

1 cup squash

Snack

Half a grapefruit

Breakfast

Oatmeal

(½ cup oats, 1 cup skim milk, 1 small banana, 1 tablespoon ground flaxseed)

Snack

1 ounce raw cashews

Lunch

No-yolk egg salad

(3 hard-boiled egg whites, 2 tablespoons hummus, sliced cucumbers, sliced tomatoes, lettuce in a whole wheat wrap)

1 peach

Snack

3 slices turkey wrapped in lettuce

Dinner

Mixed green salad with ½ cup tomatoes, ½ cup beets, 1 tablespoon ground flaxseed, salad dressing spritzer

Tofu stir-fry

(⅓ block extra-firm tofu, 2 teaspoons olive oil, 1 teaspoon low-sodium soy sauce, 1 cup sliced green and red peppers, 1 cup broccoli, 1 cup mushrooms, 1 cup bok choy, served over 1 cup brown rice)

Snack

1 cup blueberries blended in ¼ cup low-fat ricotta cheese

nutrition breakdown	grams	calories	% total
Fat	54	486	29
Carbs	249	804	47
Fiber	48	0	0
Protein	101	404	24
Total		1694	

fat-soluble vitamins	intake	RDA	% RDA
Vitamin A	1685.9 mg	800 mg	211
Vitamin D	2.45 IU	5 IU	49
Vitamin E	12.61 mg	8 mg	158
Vitamin K	636.02 mcg	65 mcg	979

trace minerals	intake	RDA	% RDA
Iron	18.4 mg	15 mg	123
Zinc	12.64 mg	12 mg	105
Selenium	98.85 mcg	55 mcg	180
Copper	3.22 mg	—	—

water-soluble vitamins	intake	RDA	% RDA
Vitamin C	450.32 mg	60 mg	751
Thiamin	1.76 mg	1.1 mg	160
Riboflavin	2.25 mg	1.1 mg	204
Vitamin B6	2.79 mg	1.3 mg	215
Vitamin B12	2.81 mcg	2.4 mcg	117
Niacin	24.46 mg	14 mg	175
Folate	614.65 mcg	400 mcg	154

major minerals	intake	RDA	% RDA
Calcium	796.49 mg	1000 mg	78
Phosphorus	1733.4 mg	700 mg	248
Magnesium	632.24 mg	310 mg	204
Sodium	2870.2 mg	—	—
Potassium	4524.1 mg	—	—

	intake	RDA	% AI
Omega-3	3.51 g	1.6 g	219

DIETARY VITAMIN SOURCES

Liver, eggs, sweet potatoes, carrots, spinach, and collard greens are excellent sources of **vitamin A**.

Excellent food sources of **vitamin C** include broccoli, bell peppers, kale, cauliflower, strawberries, lemons, Brussels sprouts, papaya, chard, cabbage, spinach, kiwifruit, cantaloupe, oranges, grapefruit, limes, tomatoes, zucchini, raspberries, asparagus, celery, pineapples, watermelon, fennel, peppermint, and parsley.

Beta-carotene can be found in concentrated amounts in a variety of foods, including sweet potatoes, carrots, kale, spinach, turnip greens, winter squash, collard greens, cilantro, fresh thyme, cantaloupe, romaine lettuce, and broccoli.

Salmon, flaxseeds, walnuts, soybeans, and halibut are excellent sources of **omega-3 fatty acids**.

Omega-6 fatty acids comprise the primary oil ingredient added to most processed foods and are found in commonly used cooking oils, including sunflower, safflower, corn, cottonseed, and soybean oils. **Gamma linolenic acid** and **linoleic acid** omega-6 fatty acids are found in the plant seed oils of evening primrose, black currant, and borage, as well as fungal oils. **Arachidonic acid** of the omega-6 series is found in egg yolks, meats (particularly organ meats), and other animal-based foods.

The best source of **omega-9 fatty acid** is olive oil. Other sources include olives, avocados, almonds, peanuts, sesame oil, pecans, pistachio nuts, cashews, hazelnuts, and macadamia nuts.

Good food sources of **alpha-lipoic acid** include spinach, broccoli, beef, yeast (particularly Brewer's yeast), and certain organ meats such as the kidney and heart.

The highest dietary sources of **coenzyme Q10** are fresh sardines and mackerel; beef, including the heart and liver; lamb; pork; and eggs. Plant sources of coenzyme Q10 include spinach, broccoli, peanuts, wheat germ, and whole grains. These foods must be raw, fresh, and unprocessed, and grown in an unpolluted environment to be considered viable sources.

GLOSSARY

acne   A skin disease in which the sebaceous glands become blocked and inflamed. Commonly affects girls and boys in puberty, but can affect people of any age.

adenosine triphosphate (ATP)   A molecule in the cellular machinery that provides energy to the cell.

alar base   The area where the nostrils attach to the cheek.

alar rim   The edge of the nostril.

alpha hydroxy acids (AHAs)   A group of mild acids that improve fine lines and wrinkles when applied regularly to the face.

amalgam   A silver-colored tooth filling containing silver and mercury.

antihelix   The undulating fold in the middle of the upper half of the ear.

antioxidants   Molecules that have extra electrons that can be used to stabilize free radicals and protect more vital unprotected molecules.

basal cell carcinoma   A skin cancer that is locally invasive and has a very small risk of spreading.

beta-carotene   A form of vitamin A and an important antioxidant.

blepharoplasty   A technique to rejuvenate the upper or lower eyelids.

Botox   A protein made by the bacteria *Clostridium botulinum* that is able to temporarily paralyze muscle.

bridge   A denture attached to the teeth on either side.

bruxism   Habitual grinding of the teeth while asleep.

carbamide peroxide   A bleaching agent used on teeth.

chemical peel   The application of acid to the face to cause skin rejuvenation.

closed rhinoplasty   A technique for cosmetic nasal surgery, whereby all incisions are inside the nose and the nasal tip is left intact.

collagen   A protein in the dermal layer of the skin that provides strength and substance to the skin. It can also be used as a filler.

columella   The area of the nasal tip that hangs down between each nasal airway.

conchal bowl   The part of the ear shaped like a bowl; the ear canal is at its base.

conformational wrinkles   Skin folds caused by bends in the body not related to muscle movement or gravity.

coronal brow lift   A surgical technique used to lift the forehead and eyebrows that results in a scar in the hair that extends from ear to ear.

corrugator supercilli   The muscle in the eyebrows that pulls the eyebrows toward the middle, producing a frowning expression.

corset platysmaplasty   A method of tightening the folds in the neck by repairing the split of the platysma.

cortisol   A steroid hormone produced by the adrenal gland that maintains many bodily functions. Skin regeneration is weakened by the increase in cortisol production associated with stress and loss of sleep.

cosmeceutical   A skin care product that has mild, unregulated amounts of active products typically regulated by the FDA.

crow's-feet   Wrinkles on the outer corner of the eye, seen while smiling or squinting and caused by the orbicularis oculi muscle.

deep plane facelift   A facelift in which the SMAS layer and the skin are lifted as a single unit to rejuvenate the face.

dentures   False teeth attached to a tray that is glued to your gums.

dermabrasion   A mechanical method of skin rejuvenation, whereby the epidermis and part of the dermis are removed by a mechanical sanding machine.

dermatitis   An inflammation of the skin. There are many different types of dermatitis.

dermis   Deep layer of skin, which provides strength and elasticity to your skin. It is also the layer that contains blood vessels, nerve endings, and hair follicles.

dynamic wrinkles   Skin folds caused by muscle movement.

elastin   A protein in the dermal layer of the skin that provides elasticity.

endoscopic brow lift   A technique to lift the forehead and eyebrows through minimal access incisions.

endoscopic midface lift   A facelift of the upper face and cheeks that is similar to or the same as the subperiosteal facelift.

epidermis   The top layer of skin that sheds dead layers outward over time and is the protective waterproof covering.

estrogen   A hormone produced in both men and woman, but most important to women and certain female bodily processes. As menopause approaches, estrogen levels drop significantly.

fluorosis   A condition affecting young children in which yellow-brown stains form on the teeth from too much fluoride in the diet.

free radical   An oxygen molecule without the desired number of necessary electrons within its structure. Because of the shortage of electrons, this molecule will take an electron from some other neighboring molecule, thereby making that molecule unstable.

frontalis   A muscle of the forehead that elevates the eyebrow.

gingivitis   An infection of the gums that can result in a receding gum line.

glabella   The area at the top of the nose between the eyebrows. This area is usually slightly recessed at the level of the upper eyelid.

glycation   The cross-linking of proteins at the cellular and genetic levels that is caused by unregulated glucose levels and insulin receptor sensitivity.

gravitational wrinkles   Skin folds caused by gravity.

gum lift   A dental treatment to correct a gummy smile by raising the gum line.

horizontal osteotomy of the mandible (HOM)   A surgical technique to shorten, lengthen, or add projection to a chin of undesirable shape. A horizontal cut is placed in the bone of the chin, and then the free segment is moved to the desired location and fixed in place.

human growth hormone (HGH)   A hormone produced by the pituitary gland that controls growth patterns in children. HGH has also been used by athletes looking for improved recuperative ability as well as those looking to stay younger looking longer.

hyaluronic acid   An important component of the dermis. This mollecule has the unique property of attracting water, similar to a sponge. It is also a primary source for cosmetic filler.

hydroquinone   A topical lotion that reduces pigmentation in the skin.

idebenone   An effective antioxidant that is demonstrated to migrate into the skin easily, thereby offering a reasonable protection for the skin.

iPLEDGE program   A governmental program deigned to educate patients on the severe risks of the acne drug Accutane in pregnancy.

keratinocytes   Skin cells in the epidermis that provide protection and hydration for your skin.

laser   A machine that focuses a single wavelength of light on a spot. A variety of dermatological laser treatments are available for hair, scar, and tattoo removal, as well as other applications.

lateral brow lift   A surgical technique to lift the lateral forehead and lateral eyebrow through a limited lateral incision within the hair of the scalp.

lifestyle lift   Skin-only facelift.

liposuction   A technique to remove fat with a vacuum-type device.

lookism   Discrimination based on physical attractiveness.

malignant melanoma   The worst form of skin cancer, which typically spreads when the lesion is of a small size. After spreading has occurred there is no adequate treatment.

melanocytes   Skin cells located at the deepest part of the epidermis that are responsible for skin pigmentation. These are also the cells that when injured can become the abnormal cells that become malignant melanoma.

metalloproteinases   Enzymes manufactured by the cells of the skin to degrade collagen and elastin. External influences, such as ultraviolet rays and pollution, can stimulate the skin cells to make more of these enzymes.

midvault   The middle one-third of the nose, comprised of cartilage. The cartilage of the side wall is called the upper lateral cartilage. Midline support is created by the septum.

nasal tip   The lower one-third of the nose.

nasojugal groove   See tear trough deformity.

Nike swoop   A slang term for the windblown look of bad plastic surgery of the face.

omega scar   A technique in facelift surgery where the scars behind the ears are placed in the fold behind the ear and then extended almost to the top of the ear and then into the hairline. This technique minimizes visibility of the scars.

open tip rhinoplasty   A cosmetic nasal surgery whereby an incision is made across the columella, as well as inside the nose, to pull back the skin of the nose to open it up for repair.

orbicularis oculi muscle   The circular muscle that surrounds the eye and closes the eyelid.

orthodontia   The practice of using braces to straighten teeth.

osteointegrated implants   Dental implants that are permanently anchored into the bone of the jaw.

otoplasty   A surgical procedure to correct for protruding or prominent ears.

peridentitis   Advanced gingivitis, which may result in tooth loss.

phytoestrogens   A dietary source of a nutrient that mimics the action of estrogen in the body.

pixie ears   A deformity of the ears whereby the earlobe is pulled tightly against the cheek as a result of facelift surgery.

platysmal bands   The inner edge of the platysma muscle in the neck. With aging, these bands hang down to create the wattle.

porcelain veneers   A technique used to repair chipped or cracked teeth in which a coating of porcelain is bonded to the front and sides of the tooth.

pretrichial brow lift   A surgical technique to lift the forehead and eyebrow with an incision at the hairline.

proanthocyanidin   An effective antioxidant that is demonstrated to migrate into the skin easily, thereby offering a reasonable protection for the skin.

Retin-A   A derivative of vitamin A that is useful against acne as well as fine lines and wrinkles.

rhinoplasty   A surgical procedure to make the nose more cosmetically appealing and/ or improve airway function.

root canal   The process of removing the soft root of a tooth when it is infected or dead.

SMAS facelift　A facelift that moves the skin and SMAS as two separate layers. Different variations of this techniques have been done for more than 30 years.

squamous cell carcinoma　A skin cancer that is typically locally invasive and will only spread outside the local area if untreated for a long period of time.

subcutaneous tissue　The layer of fat and nerves just below the dermal layer of the skin that adds volume and contour to your skin.

submusculoaponeurotic system (SMAS)　The layer of muscle and fascia below the skin of the face.

subperiosteal facelift　A facelift that lifts the tissue from a surgical plane just above the bones of the face.

sunscreen　A chemical applied to the skin designed to absorb the dangerous ultraviolet rays of the sun and thereby protect the cells from such damage.

tear trough deformity　Also called nasojugal groove. The depression that extends from the inner corner of the eye, below the eye, and across the cheek.

thread lift　A surgical technique whereby a barbed wire is passed through the cheeks and the cheeks are suspended by the barbs to create a minimally invasive cheek lift.

tip delivery rhinoplasty　A cosmetic nasal surgery technique where the incisions are inside the nose. The nasal tip cartilage is partially pulled outside the nose, then trimmed and manipulated and placed back inside the nose.

turbinates　Specialized mucous membranes within the nasal airway that filter, humidify, and control the rate of airflow inside the nose.

turkey gobbler release　A simple method to put multiple small releasing incisions in the platysmal bands to create a smooth neck contour.

ultraviolet radiation　A type of energy that comes from the sun along with normal daylight. This form of energy is divided into groups, with the UV "A" and UV "B" rays being most important to skin. The "A" rays are present outdoors throughout the year and from dawn until dusk. This group of rays causes aging and increased risk for cancer. The "B" rays are prevalent during the summer months, and only during midday. These rays cause sunburns and also contribute to an increased risk of skin cancer.

vertical submental skin excision   A surgical technique to remove excess neck skin through direct skin excision on the neck.

vitamin C   A water-soluble vitamin/antioxidant in both oral form and topical creams (L-ascorbic acid). Also, an essential building block for wound healing and collagen strength.

vitamin E   An important antioxidant.

INDEX

nasal. *See* nose

nasojugal grooves, 140

neck, 121–127, 131, 224

neck lift, 126

New Age skin care, 37–41

Nike swoop, 103

nonablative laser treatments, 67

noninvasive skin care procedures, 56–59

nose, 149–170
  anatomy, 152–160
  costs, 167–168
  ethnicity and balance, 150–152
  ideals, 107
  rhinoplasties, 160–167, 224

nose
  self-assessment, 169

nostril shapes, 151

nutrition. *See* diet (eating habits)

O

office tone and ambience, 211

omega-3 fatty acids, 36, 247

omega scar, 127, 253

open tip rhinoplasty, 163–165, 167

orthodontia, 183–184

osteointegrated implants, 187

otoplasty, 189–193, 224

oval face, hair design for, 90

overselling surgery, 119

over-the-counter products, 79–81

P

pain relievers, 219

parent responsibilities. *See* teens

patchy hair loss, 196–197

peels, 57–59

peer pressure, 228

permanent fillers, 64–65

phenol peels, 58–59

philosophy, surgeon, 210–211

physical exercise, 234–235

physical sunscreens, 81–82

phytoestrogens, 40

piercing (ears), 192–193

pigment changes, 70–71

pixie ears, 103

plastic surgeon selection, 101–103, 207–214
  initial consultation, 229–230, 238
  for rhinoplasty, 160–161

platysma bands, 122–123

platysmaplasty, 123–125

pollution, 32–33

poly-L-lactic acid, 63

porcelain veneers (teeth), 186

positive attitude, 231–232

postauricular scarring, 104

postoperative recovery. *See* recovery

preparing for surgery, 215–224

prescriptions, for surgery, 219

presurgical testing, 216

pretrichial brow lift, 143–144

products. *See* beauty products

progesterone levels, 40

Propecia, 201

proteins, 38–39

protruding ears, 189–192

psychological components of surgery, 225

R

Radiesse. *See* calcium hydroxyapatite crystals

recovery, 222–224

after lower face surgery, 129–130, 224
  after rhinoplasty, 167, 224
  otoplasty, 192, 224
  preparing for, 216–217

redraping, 124

removing tattoos, 69–70

Restylane. *See* hyaluronic acid (HA)

Retin-A, 46–47, 53, 71, 235, 254

retinoids, 52–54

rhinophyma, 158

rhinoplasties, 160–167, 224. *See also* nose
  costs, 167–168

round face, hair design for, 91

S

salicylic acid, 55, 83

scalp reduction, 203

scar and scab care, 222–223

scars at ears, 104

sclerotherapy, 69

Sculptra. *See* poly-L-lactic acid

self-assessment
  lower face, 131–132
  nose, 169

septum, 156–157

serum glucose levels, 38–39

sideburn, loss of, 103

silicone beads, 64–65

silicone droplets, 65

skin, 21–41, 235–236. *See also* sun protection
  aging effects, 44–45, 96–100, 134
  anatomy, 22–24
  bleaches, 56
  health basics, 25–33

skin, *cont.*